Residential Work with the Elderly

First published in 1977, *Residential Work with the Elderly* brings together theoretical and practical approaches of relevance to providing care for older people in residential homes and long-stay geriatric hospitals. He describes the kinds of use to which institutional care is commonly put, the effects of institutional living on individual residents and the ageing process. He also examines ways of using such care to the benefit of both individuals and the resident group, so that new, improved ways may be found of helping older people in care.

Intended principally for residential workers in homes for the elderly, the book is also designed for nurses and other workers involved in long-term hospital care for older people. It will also be of value to those involved in day-care and special housing provision for the elderly.

Residential Work with the Elderly

C. Paul Brearley

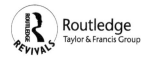

Routledge
Taylor & Francis Group

First published in 1977
By Routledge & Kegan Paul

This edition first published in 2022 by Routledge
4 Park Square, Milton Park, Abingdon, Oxon, OX14 4RN
and by Routledge
605 Third Avenue, New York, NY 10017

Routledge is an imprint of the Taylor & Francis Group, an informa business

Publisher's Note
The publisher has gone to great lengths to ensure the quality of this reprint but points
out that some imperfections in the original copies may be apparent.

Disclaimer
The publisher has made every effort to trace copyright holders and welcomes
correspondence from those they have been unable to contact.

A Library of Congress record exists under ISBN: 0710085877

ISBN: 978-1-032-47261-4 (hbk)
ISBN: 978-1-003-38530-1 (ebk)
ISBN: 978-1-032-47262-1 (pbk)

Book DOI 10.4324/9781003385301

Residential work with the elderly

C. Paul Brearley
Senior Lecturer in Social Work,
University College of North Wales,
Bangor

Routledge & Kegan Paul
London, Henley and Boston

First published in 1977
by Routledge & Kegan Paul Ltd
39 Store Street,
London WC1E 7DD,
Broadway House,
Newtown Road,
Henley-on-Thames,
Oxon RG9 1EN and
9 Park Street,
Boston, Mass. 02108, USA
Set in 10 on 11pt English
and printed in Great Britain by
The Lavenham Press Limited
Lavenham, Suffolk

British Library Cataloguing in Publication Data

Brearley, Christopher Paul

Residential work with the elderly — (Library of social work).

1. Old age homes
I. Title II. Series
362.6'15   HV1451

ISBN 0-7100-8587-7
ISBN 0-7100-8588-5 Pbk
ISSN 0305-4381

Contents

Contents

Preface

Working with the elderly has often been seen as unattractive and depressing by members of the professional groups concerned with meeting their needs for health and social services. Similarly work in residential homes and in continuing-care hospitals for the elderly has usually been regarded by nurses, doctors and social workers as unrewarding. Certainly there have been relatively few attempts to develop treatment and caring approaches in these areas, and training, too, has been limited. In spite of this superficially negative-seeming picture there are many positives to be found in the current practice of nurses and residential workers.

It has been my intention, in writing this book, to bring together, in an organised way, some of the ideas, concepts and skills which seem to be relevant to the field of work. I do not wish to suggest that the work is easy or that change will come about without hard and careful effort. I do think, however, that existing knowledge and skills can be effectively organised and that it is at the very least possible to look for new and improved ways of helping older people in care. Work with the elderly can be interesting, worth-while and successful.

My thanks are due to all those colleagues, residents and patients who have given help and support in the development of my ideas on this subject, and to my wife for her help and comments while I have been writing this book.

Chapter one

Introduction

Residential care for the elderly grew largely out of Poor Law development. In recent years geriatric medicine has emerged as a recognisable branch of medicine but both hospital and residential services for the elderly have suffered from being provided in outdated buildings. The pressure of demand on all services for the elderly in the community and in institutional care is increasing as the population grows and population structure changes. Health and social services are failing to meet the demands that are being made on them and there is an increasing gap between consumer needs and the extent of provisions to meet these needs. The elderly, until recently, have been at the end of the queue for resources, partly because of society's general attitudes to ageing, partly because of the low value and status accorded to work with older people, and partly because the elderly themselves often accept a low self-evaluation and are inclined to make few demands.

The approaches to improving services and to closing the gap between needs and provisions will have to be on many levels. The priority for the majority of older people will be the provision of services in their own homes. Studies vary slightly in their estimates but it seems that between 4 per cent and 5 per cent of people over 65 are in some form of institutional care—hospital, local authority, private or voluntarily-run accommodation. If 95 per cent of the elderly live, and wish to continue living, in their own homes then they should be able to receive the kind of domiciliary support services which will make their quality of life as satisfying as possible. Some older people will not be able to live at home and may need a period of temporary or permanent care in an institutional setting. If they are to live contented, satisfying lives in enclosed, communal groups attention must be given to the appropriate use of existing facilities, as well as to the extension of resources.

Introduction

Only relatively few residential workers have a recognised qualification in residential work, in comparison to social workers in the community. A working-party discussion document of the Central Council for Education and Training in Social Work (CCETSW, 1973) suggested a 'worrying figure of 62% of staff without any form of qualification or training'. Exact figures are difficult to reproduce in relation to care for the elderly, because nursing qualifications have usually been acceptable for posts in residential work with the elderly. Work in long-term institutional care for the elderly has been of low status because of a feeling that it is concerned mainly with people in a state of pre-death: homes and long-stay geriatric hospitals have been seen by staff, residents and community as ante-rooms to death. The lower status of residential workers has been emphasised by the fact that admissions are usually arranged by field workers. Involvement of the residential worker in decisions on admission is frequently minimal, and sometimes non-existent. The comparatively low status is reflected in the treatment of residential workers. There is no real career structure in residential work with the elderly: this is particularly difficult to assess because nursing staff are quite likely to transfer from hospital to residential care and it is hard for them to measure success or improved status. Added to this is the lack of an adequate pay structure, and insufficient professional support and back-up facilities. Since the job has been perceived as having limited attractions recruitment is difficult and staffing levels are low. Many workers find themselves working long hours under stressful conditions: if they live on the premises there is no escape from demands.

The position is aggravated in some situations by the conflict of objectives that may exist in general and individual terms. A local-authority social services department usually has a long waiting list for admission to care: the residential worker is made aware of pressure from outside by anxious relatives of older people waiting for admission, by field social workers and by administrative staff. This can only cause stress for the residential worker, who must provide a continuing life for residents but feels under pressure to create vacancies for new admissions. Field social workers may have unrealistic expectations of the kind of care or treatment situation that is available in a home and raise additional pressures for the residential worker by implicit and explicit suggestions that impossible objectives should be achieved. Other problems may arise from the failure of field workers—under many different pressures of work-loads themselves—to follow up older people after admission to care, or to provide sufficient preparation and information before admission.

This book will look at some of the problems of communal living,

2

at some of the special needs of older people in care, at ways of improving standards and styles of care, as well as at the relationships between residential and field workers and ways in which these might be improved to provide a better consumer service.

Availability and nature of care

Although institutional care for the elderly will be examined in a fairly generalised way, the actual range of care is often very different in nature and extent. It is important to be aware of some of the differences between the available forms of accommodation as well as the similarities.

Historical aspects

The early history of provision for the elderly in this country is one of voluntary care, and especially care provided by the church. Monastic infirmary almshouses represented the main provision for the elderly until the Reformation. When Henry VIII instituted the dissolution of the monasteries, numbers of the sick and infirm were made homeless and destitute. The Poor Law Act of 1601 placed the responsibility for care of the needy on each parish and for the next three-and-a-half centuries care was provided in a mixed workhouse environment in which young, old, blind, mentally ill, sick and disabled people were cared for together. From the end of the eighteenth century the parishes increasingly adopted a system of supplementing low wages on a scale regulated by the price of bread, and this eventually had the effect of reducing the ordinary working man to the position of pauper. The Poor Law Amendment Act of 1834 grouped parishes into Unions under the supervision of Boards of Guardians. The Act also made the workhouses, which by then had been established in most places, a general provision: outdoor relief (relief outside the workhouse) could only be given to the sick, the elderly, widows and children, and relief to the able-bodied only in the workhouse. The implication, therefore, was that with an atmosphere of strict discipline the able-bodied poor would be discouraged from applying for help and driven to stay away from the workhouses. Although there were some charitably maintained almshouses, most institutional care for older people was based on a utilitarian attitude to the undeserving poor.

In the latter part of the last century as much as a third of the population had to resort to poor relief at some period during their lives. In 1908 the first old age pension was introduced and in 1925 this was extended by the principle of social insurance. Payment to the elderly then became a return from contributions rather than a charitable payment from the state. In 1929 the Local Government Act transferred the powers of the Boards of Guardians to the county and county borough councils, who were permitted to reclassify some of the institutions as hospitals. Changes and upheavals in traditional social relationships during the Second World War exposed a great deal of need, and new attitudes led to the establishment of the National Health Service, and residential care was developed following the National Assistance Act in 1948.

In the immediate post-war years and the early 1950s shortages of building materials and government restrictions on capital expenditure hindered the building of new establishments. The elderly continued to be cared for in 'upgraded' workhouse institutions and in converted premises—usually large, older houses with steep stairs, often with big rooms sleeping five, six or more residents. In 1954 a review of provision of old people's homes was undertaken, leading to the recommendation that homes of up to sixty residents should be built, especially where demand was heavy and sites few in the more populated areas (Ministry of Health, 1955). At the same time other studies (Department of Health (Scotland), 1953; Boucher, 1957) indicated the shortage of places in residential accommodation and there were also practical difficulties of determining whether the chronically sick elderly should be cared for in hospital or residential accommodation. The ministry took the view, however, that long-term building plans should not begin until more was known about the effect of the development of geriatric care on overall need (Phillips Committee, 1954). The Phillips Committee emphasised the need for the development of domiciliary care and the importance of people in institutional care retaining a community orientation. In 1957 a further Circular (Ministry of Health, 1957) approved these views and made an attempt to redefine the distinctions between hospital and residential care.

After the 1959 Mental Health Act local authorities had power to provide residential accommodation for the mentally infirm and this, combined with a lifting of capital restriction, encouraged an increase in building until Townsend's attack on the emphasis on residential provision in *The Last Refuge* (1962).

The issue of who should provide continuous nursing care for those elderly people who needed it still remained. The increasing emphasis in residential accommodation was on the needs of the frail elderly and this brought out additional issues about the need to employ people with nursing qualifications, and night attendants. By the mid-1960s the major emphasis was being placed on care in the community through improved and extended domiciliary health and welfare services. In 1968 a further government social survey (Harris, 1968) indicated that many older people are admitted to care because

4

of unsuitable alternative accommodation. A ministry memorandum (Ministry of Health, 1965) to local authorities and hospitals set out broad categories of older people for whom they might normally expect to have to provide accommodation. It also suggested that the right way to deal with those who were wrongly placed was to accept the *status quo* for those already in care but to try to avoid wrong placement, in the future, by joint planning.

The broad development of institutional care has, then, moved from an entirely charitable provision, through a philosophy of strict workhouse provision designed to discourage rather than care, to the post-war developments. Since the National Assistance Act residential care has been through several stages: immediately after the Act provision was in adapted accommodation, from 1954 to about 1960-2 it was in larger, purpose-built homes, and from the early 1960s developments have tended to be in the form of smaller homes. The emphasis of the 1970s has been on domiciliary services, and residential care is increasingly being seen as a community resource to be used as part of a treatment approach to elderly people in need.

The context of care—hospital and residential home

Hospitals are concerned primarily with treatment of illness and disease and with returning the individual to a state of good health and to his normal community roles and with limiting the disabling effects of impairment. Long-term hospital care will have to be provided for some elderly patients who are very infirm or suffering from chronic illness and need a degree of nursing care that is unavailable elsewhere. Normally this means that social support networks in the community are inadequate or non-existent: most families do provide good, concerned care for their elderly relatives, sometimes to the point of exhaustion and collapse. Those hospitals and wards that provide long-term care share similar goals to those of residential accommodation, of meeting individual needs for a degree of stimulation, satisfaction and contentment.

The basic task is to provide patients and residents with an adequate quality of life. The nature of adequacy will vary and it should not be forgotten that patients in geriatric hospitals are often extremely frail and frequently are both physically and mentally infirm. Although the same can be said of some residents in old people's homes there can be no doubt that elderly patients make heavier demands for physical care on staff and this will affect the nature of the relationship. In some senses expectations of the hospital are different from those of the residential home: the sick role contains an acceptance that the patient will give up certain activities and be dependent whereas admission to an old people's home may often be seen as 'defeat' and 'failure' and contain punitive elements. These and similar expectations and attitudes will create differences in the ways in which workers and elderly people in care relate to each other.

Nevertheless institutional care has many common factors in the nature of the social systems involved and the pressures that are created for staff and residents. Most important, individuals have the same rights to respect and similar needs for flexible, individual care in either hospital or home. The terms 'resident' and 'patient' are often used in the same context throughout this book and this reflects the similarities in institutional pressures and individual needs within the communal group. The differences in the hospital and residential situation (especially the greater degree of disability, the more obvious treatment functions, the larger group and the more formalised structure of the former) should also be borne in mind.

Sheltered housing

Sheltered housing or grouped dwellings for older people is specially designed accommodation provided specifically for elderly tenants, often with a warden employed in a supportive role. A few authorities began to build such schemes in the early post-war years but it was not until 1957 that the Ministry of Housing and Local Government (1957) began to encourage local authorities to develop schemes and offered advice on planning and design. Development of schemes has progressed steadily ever since and this form of provision is becoming increasingly popular.

Since it is a relatively new service there is little information about the kinds of people who live in sheltered housing or about the effects of such accommodation on tenants. There seem to be a number of goals implicit in the policies for selection of tenants—the prolongation of life, the prevention of the use of more expensive services, etc. (Willcocks, 1975). Nevertheless there is insufficient overall agreement on goals and a lack of available research findings on which to base a clarification of objectives. Several writers have pointed to the close relationship between sheltered housing and residential accommodation with the implication that the former might, or should, replace the latter in the long run. At the present time there appears to be less chance of the old person in special housing moving to more intensive forms of care than there is for older people from other community situations. A study in Devon (Boldy, Abel and Carter, 1973) suggested that for most tenants 'grouped dwellings are currently providing a setting within which it is expected that their care requirements may be met until death'.

Clearly there is a growth in the provision of sheltered housing and the emphasis is shifting from residential care for some older people at least. The relevance of the growth of such provision for this discussion lies particularly in the need for a more clearly defined role for the wardens of the schemes and for training for the wardens. A working party report (Age Concern, 1974, p. 5) suggested that:

> the warden plays a large part in determining the quality of life in grouped schemes, and has a vital contribution to make in their day-to-day running. Therefore it is essential that wardens be given the opportunity to increase their background knowledge and to refine their skills in order to carry out their task more effectively.

The report goes on to propose a course of training for wardens that would give knowledge of physiological and sociological ageing processes, of human needs (physiological needs, security, social needs, self-esteem, growth and human potential), of the nature and value of roles and relationships, of interpersonal communication, and of services and facilities, home safety and maintenance of buildings and equipment.

The task of the warden has many elements in common with that of the residential worker. The main area of functioning is, of course, concerned with creating an environment with basic components of comfort and safety. To achieve this the warden will be involved in ensuring that the property is physically in order, with giving advice and information to tenants, with providing emergency services and generally encouraging individual satisfaction within a secure, comfortable material environment. The warden will also have a part to play with regard to the tenant group as a whole—with the encouragement of friendship, mutual help, and a sense of shared experience through group activities. If these functions are to be carried out effectively the warden will need support from a number of directions. A recognition of the warden's need for a separate life requires administrative and practical help for holiday and weekend relief, etc. At least as important is the need for other caring groups in the community to work with the warden in providing the best environment and help for the individual tenant. The administrative split between housing, health and social services has too often led to wardens feeling isolated and unsupported—as well as frequently leaving them carrying inappropriate burdens of nursing and domestic responsibilities.

I would suggest, then, that the task of the warden in sheltered housing could be very similar to that of the residential worker. Although this book is not specifically aimed at wardens in grouped housing schemes for the elderly it will, hopefully, offer some ideas and guidance appropriate to many of their tasks.

Introduction

Patterns of care

Why do people go into residential accommodation? Several studies have examined reasons for application for care, the first important major study being the government survey *Social Welfare for the Elderly* (Harris, 1968). Two subsequent studies are also of particular interest: a study of *The Elderly in Residential Care* (Carstairs and Morrison, 1971) and *Care of the Elderly,* an exercise in cost benefit analysis in the care of the elderly (Wager, 1972).

Harris found that the majority of residents said that they wanted to go into a home. The most usual reason for admission was because the person was unable to care for himself in his own home, and often this stage was reached immediately after a spell of illness. A number of residents were found to have applied because their doctors had recommended it on the grounds that they might fall, or that they would be in danger alone at night. Another group were those who did not want to be a burden to their children: these residents were likely to have initiated the application themselves, as were those who came as a result of family quarrels. About 7 per cent of residents studied by Harris went into care more because of a wish for companionship than because they could not manage physically outside, and about 2 per cent got into financial difficulties. Harris also suggested that a high proportion of residents have to go into residential accommodation because they have nowhere to live, quite often as a result of selling homes or giving up tenancies on admission to hospital. Also in connection with housing needs she found that relatively few adequately housed council house tenants applied for admission to a home but that of the elderly who lived as boarders, or in rooms or lodgings, rather more were admitted than might be expected from the total numbers of elderly living in such conditions. Inadequate housing provision seems to be a key factor for many applications from the evidence of this study.

Carstairs and Morrison found that, of residents in all the homes they studied, about two-thirds came direct from the community. Just over a third (34 per cent) of all residents had been living alone before coming in (a study by Bennett et al. (1968) found as many as 45 per cent lived alone before admission), and another 28 per cent had been with friends or relatives. Almost 20 per cent came from hospitals and 5 per cent had been in hotels, lodgings or boarding houses. They also found some movement between residential homes: 9 per cent of residents came from other forms of residential care.

Wager suggested that the need for care of half the applicants (51 per cent) arose from inability to look after themselves, or from anticipated inability to care for themselves, the rest of the applications being accounted for by loneliness (8 per cent), difficulties in relationships in the household (8 per cent), accommodation problems (4 per cent), or a combination of factors. This study also found a relationship between living situation and the cause of application: old people living alone, for instance, accounted for 55 per cent of those applying for reasons of incapacity, and 80 per cent of those who appeared to be applying in case of future incapacity lived alone. On the other hand all but one of the nineteen applications arising from accommodation problems or homelessness were from old people living with others.

The significant factors in applications for residential care seem, as might be expected, to be incapacity for self-care, inadequate or unsuitable accommodation, and to a lesser extent loneliness or difficult relationships with others living in the same household. With this background to admission what are the characteristics of residents living in homes? Harris suggests that, in the main, people who are admitted are women, single or widowed and at least 75 years of age. Carstairs and Morrison found the mean age of residents was 79·8 years, compared with a figure of 73·4 years for the elderly population as a whole; over 30 per cent of residents were 85 years old or more (women tending to be older than men). Dependency of residents was measured in an attempt to relate staffing levels to dependency levels of residents and it was found that age was an important influence on physical and mental condition: generally, successive age-groups show a declining proportion of fully fit individuals.

More than 60 per cent of residents were mentally alert, slightly more were fully mobile, and almost 80 per cent always continent. Carstairs and Morrison also found some important differences between local-authority, private and voluntary accommodation. Some 85 per cent of residents in voluntary homes were fully capable and only 5 per cent had complete incapacity, compared with figures of 67 per cent and 11 per cent for local-authority homes. They showed that over a third of all residents show no impairment whatsoever, and a further 17 per cent show only mild impairment.

Clearly some residents do not have a physical need for residential accommodation. Harris suggested that most residents are quite content to be living in care but Slater (1968) has demonstrated that satisfactory adjustment in residential accommodation is linked to higher degrees of disability. It may well be that some residents are fit for discharge and are sufficiently motivated to seek other forms of accommodation in the community. Harris, however, found that of the sixty-six residents in all the areas studied who wanted to return to the community, apparently only twenty-five could manage even if suitable housing was available.

What, then, happens to people in residential accommodation in terms of discharge opportunities? Carstairs and Morrison found an annual turnover of 36 per cent of the resident population; half the total number of discharges were deaths. Of the live discharges the great majority were to hospital or other forms of residential care. Nevertheless 13 per cent of live discharges were of people going to live with relatives, and another 5 per cent went to live alone. An increasing number of residential places are used for short-term provision and this accounts for some changing patterns of discharge. It is important to bear in mind that if even 5 per cent of residents are discharged from institutional care altogether that will release 5 beds in every 100. For most local authorities that would mean at least the resident population of one home in a year—about fifty people. If beds can be released by increased turnover then a better service can be offered to the whole community.

A continuum of care

In order to offer such a service it is essential to recognise the interdependence of all the services that are available. The caring continuum is not necessarily a downward slope from community to residential accommodation to hospital to death. It may be a circular route from community to hospital, to residential care, back home again, or any variation of available services. The key concept in an effective use of services is flexibility of approach.

It is clear from many studies done in a wide range of contexts that the divisions of consumer need are very blurred. Many very disabled and infirm elderly people are being cared for in the community by their families. Some less infirm older people are in long-stay hospital wards, unable to return home because they have never had, or no longer have, any family to care for them. Others have sold their homes or have given up tenancies or could not store furniture, and so they have no way out. Yet others are waiting for transfer to a residential home but cannot be moved because of lack of a 'suitable' vacancy, perhaps because of incontinence, or simply because they have had to wait for so long that they have sunk into a state of apathy and disinterest and their condition has deteriorated so they are no longer fit enough for discharge. A rather similar picture exists in residential situations. Some residents need more care than the home would normally offer but residential workers are reluctant to send them to hospital because they may have lived in the home for years. Others were admitted to care after deteriorating through lack of support, money and adequate housing: with good food, companionship, warmth and comfort they improve to such a degree that they could cope in sheltered housing but are unable to find the housing or the furniture to fill it.

Artificial, essentially administrative, barriers may also exist, hindering progress through the caring system. Sometimes sick people in residential care can only be moved to hospital in exchange for a patient waiting for transfer: this form of body-swapping leads to hurried transfers, often leaving the elderly people concerned confused, disorientated, dissatisfied and far from home. Local problems of distrust between workers in the field, in hospital, and in the homes may also build up as a result of a few mistakes or mishandled exchanges. Elitist thinking on the part of groups of workers is also inclined to lead to splitting up of functions: elitist approaches inevitably leave the elderly consumer at the bottom of the pile. Until administrative barriers can be made more flexible in policy terms, and in terms of worker relationships, the continuum of caring approaches cannot be used appropriately to meet individual need in the correct way. Each elderly person should be at the right place in the system for his own needs, at the right time. One way to encourage this is for workers to be able to function as a team to put consumer need before their own divisive needs.

The report of a working party on residential work as a part of social work (CCETSW, 1974) argued that social workers share a common knowledge base, relating to human behaviour (individual and social) and drawing on other disciplines such as psychology, psychiatry, medicine and sociology. In arguing this they acknowledge that social-work practice in particular settings requires additional knowledge, but emphasise the generic basis of social work. When workers in all the caring professions concerned with the elderly begin to recognise the similarities of their work, rather than the differences, the continuum of care may become a useful reality.

Attitudes and the elderly

An important element in the development of services for older people is that of attitudes held by the community in general terms to 'old people', as well as the attitudes of professionals involved with the elderly, and the attitudes of the elderly themselves to their needs, to being old, and to the kind of care that is provided for them.

Some population trends are important. There are more old people now in relation to the number of people available to meet their needs for care: there are proportionately more children as well as more older people in comparison to those of working age. This does not mean that people are living to be older than in previous centuries but means that more people are living to be old because of better medical care—especially the control of infectious diseases such as tuberculosis, etc. In a sense old people are survivors: they have overcome a large number of hazards to reach old age and by implication have particular strengths. This was much more the case in previous centuries when the few people who reached old age really were much more resilient (and lucky) than the majority of the population. One implication of this trend is that we have not just a larger proportion of older people but a larger proportion of people who are very old. On the whole it is the very old and especially those over 85 years who are more likely to be infirm and to require support services. In addition to this, women are likely to live longer than men and many older women are also widowed: the widowed are also a group who make increased demands on services.

There are other implications of the changing population structure that are relevant to providing health and social services. When older people reach the age of 80 or 85 their children, who are the ones who usually provide support and care, will be reaching later middle age themselves and will be less able to care. It has traditionally been the unmarried daughter who often stayed at home to care for her parents in their old age: changes in expectations and in the male-female balance are likely to remove this form of support as well. Similarly, married daughters are more likely to wish to go out to work and the choice between a regular addition to the family income and caring for ageing parents will be a difficult one. These and other similar changes influence the rate and nature of demand on the caring continuum. Changes in the population structure may bring long-term changes in society's attitudes to the elderly and the appropriateness of care.

Industrialised societies have no clear role that can be recognised as the role of the 'old person'. Old age is socially and often rigidly defined by retirement but obviously no radical changes take place at the age of 65 that change an individual from 'being middle aged' to 'being old'. One common view of old age represents older people as the victims of our society in which a number of conditions exist and which affect the ways in which older people are perceived. It is suggested that there are limited opportunities for learning how to behave as an old person and since little value is placed on the skills and wisdom of the older worker (except, perhaps, in political roles!)—in contrast to pre-industrialised societies—there is little motivation to learn as long as it can be avoided. Rosow (1967) has suggested that although older people do have some opportunities to interact with others of their own age they are much more likely to identify their peers as old than they are to see themselves as old. The more active they remain the less likely they are to identify themselves as old, but the less active they are the fewer opportunities they have for learning how to behave as old. Rosow argues that the result of the various pressures on the older person is a confusion about how older people should behave in the minds of all concerned and this role-ambiguity may lead many people to fall back on stereotyped attitudes.

Some common stereotypes are easily identifiable: older people are rigid and inflexible; older people are irritable and self-centred; older people are self-assertive and dominating; older people tend to return to the past and refuse to try new things. There are also more positive stereotypes: patience, tolerance, an ability to listen, wisdom, loyalty, hard work and restraint are all suggested as stereotyped ideals of what old people ought to be able to give (Gilhome, 1974). The danger of these stereotypes is that people who grow older may have no other yardstick of behaviour and accept the stereotyped expectations. They may feel that to try out new things is undignified, or that they have a right to be self-centred or controlling. Some of these behaviour patterns will be found in some older people and their validity is discussed in more detail later. What is clear is that all people have a right to grow old in the way that they have grown up—in an individual way in response to their own genetic inheritance and internal environment against their own individual, particular, environmental background of experience.

One view of old age sees it as social deprivation (Harris, 1972): the older person is deprived of his economic portion in society and his work-related roles and he is deprived of an active family role. Instead of being the breadwinner he becomes dependent: a recipient rather than a provider. He loses the authority that his social knowledge gave him as he is left behind by social changes. The greater dependence on the family and the wider social deprivations are unwelcome. Harris suggests that the position of the old can be 'understood in terms of their participation in exchange relationships in both society and family. Whether or not deprivation occurs depends on the extent to which, in both spheres, the old can continue to give as well as to receive. Loss of opportunity to give is itself a deprivation.'

A rather similar approach sees the problems of ageing as problems of decreasing power resources (Dowd, 1975). Older people are represented as increasingly unable to enter into balanced exchange relations with other groups with whom they interact: the power of the older person relative to the exchange partner increasingly deteriorates. In this imbalanced exchange relationship the older person is compelled to exchange compliance for continuing sustenance.

These arguments rest on an assumed compliant position of the elderly as a group and the evidence that the elderly can be viewed or view themselves in such homogeneous terms is limited. In general terms some elements are evident. Stereotypes may be common but research findings suggest that the majority of older people are

Introduction

closely involved with other people in their social environment and locality. On the other hand for a fairly substantial minority problems arise as a result of their being demonstrably less involved than when they were younger. There is also a difference between the ageing process as experienced by individuals and the position of old people as a group. Our society seems to have little clear conception of the role of the old person and a degree of confusion and role-ambiguity is overlaid on the pattern of individual experience. Most people seem to experience ageing as fairly satisfactory: it is those who for a variety of reasons are unable to achieve the level of social involvement and activity they need and want—the compulsorily disengaged—who are likely to present problems.

The confusion of society and of the elderly themselves over what behaviour is appropriate to old age, and towards older people, exists also for the professional worker in providing care. Social workers, for example, are much more likely to give negative stereotypes about the elderly than about other client groups, and similarly medical students are likely to produce negative views, characterising old people as disagreeable, inactive, economically burdensome, and dull (Blank, 1971). A study of Social Service Department workers (Neill et al., 1973) also found that social workers placed the elderly with the mentally handicapped at the end of their list of priorities of satisfying groups to work with. This reluctance to work with the elderly is certainly related to an often realistic feeling that progress must be limited with older people, that the inevitable end result is death, and that older people are often depressed and, for some workers, depressing. It may also be linked to the workers' feelings about old age and death: unresolved fears and anxieties about ageing and death may affect the ability to work effectively with older people. Another real problem is the lack of resources: a good deal of work with older people is concerned with meeting practical needs and if resources are not available this will create frustrations for the worker.

Summary

There is a gap between the needs of older people and the availability of health and social services. A good deal of effort in recent years has been devoted to the increase of resources to meet the need and especially the need for domiciliary resources. In addition to the increase in availability of resources it is also important to think about improving the use of existing resources. If all the caring resources for the elderly can be seen as a continuum or interlinked circle of provision, each individual can then be fully assessed and placed according to his individual need.

This book is concerned with the place of residential care in the totality of provision for the elderly and with the appropriate use and handling of residential resources to meet individual needs. These objectives are clouded at present by confusion of attitudes to 'old age' or 'the elderly' and by the low status of both residential care and work with the elderly. A look at the special needs of older people in the setting of residential accommodation and at the common knowledge base of social work in various situations may help to clarify some of these aspects. In considering older people in residential care the similarities between continuing-care hospitals and old people's homes will tend to be emphasised but the differences between the two contexts should not be forgotten.

Chapter two

Aspects of communal living

In order to gain some insights into the need for different kinds of approaches to the provision of long-term care of individual older people it will be important to look first of all at the general effects of living in enclosed group situations. The word 'institutionalisation' has acquired many negative connotations, partly associated with confusion over the meaning and appropriate use of the term. It is possible to disentangle some of its uses and to clarify some of the real effects of institutional living.

Institutionalisation

(i) What characterises an institution?

Residential institutions, whether hospitals, prisons or old people's homes have an internal life of their own: each institution has an organised social system which is maintained by all those people who function within it. There have been several studies of residential institutions for adults which have examined the characteristic processes within institutions (Stanton and Schwartz, 1954; Belknap, 1956; Greenblatt, Levinson and Williams, 1957; Caudill, 1958). Most of these studies have tended to examine processes of interaction within the organisational system, often taking a descriptive approach.

Goffman (1961) has made a very important contribution to the sociological study of residential institutions as organisations in terms of their caring functions within a wider society. In *Asylums*, he suggests that institutions have an encompassing, total character which is symbolised by barriers to interaction with external society. Often, he contends, these barriers are built into the structure of the institution in the form of high walls, locked doors, etc., but they may equally be implicit in other restrictions on departure and outside

16

contacts. He lists the total institutions in our society in five rough groupings. First, there are those established to care for people who are both incapable and felt to be harmless (e.g. the old, the blind, etc.). Second, there are institutions caring for incapable people who may present a threat to the community (e.g. psychiatric hospitals), and third, there are institutions to contain those who present intentional dangers (e.g. prisons). Other institutions are established in order to pursue working tasks better, and finally some are designed as retreats from the world.

Goffman's concept of the total institution has several central features. All aspects of life—sleeping, eating, working and playing— are carried out in the same place under the same control: all daily living activities have to take place in the company of others who tend to be treated alike; all phases of a day's activities are tightly scheduled; and finally all activities are brought together in one plan to fulfil the official aims of the institution. Some of these generalised ideas can be applied to long-term care for the elderly and the negative connotations examined. It should, of course, be borne in mind that Goffman was dealing with an ideal type, and individual institutions must be viewed with rather more flexibility. A number of central elements are apparent:

Ritualisation and standardisation of task performance and of behaviour is usual. A lack of staffing resources is commonly given as the reason for having a fixed schedule for task performance. The hospital beds must all be made before breakfast, so all patients must be up and dressed by 7.30 a.m.: domestic staff in an old people's home follow a rigid programme to fit in their cleaning duties before giving out the morning drink, so residents cannot use a sitting room until after the carpet has been swept at 9.00 a.m. every day; examples are numerous.

Rigidity and inflexibility are by no means restricted to staff behaviour patterns. Many residents in homes and in hospitals for the elderly insist on having their own chair in the lounge and dining room. Any violation of their territorial rights is greeted with strong reactions. In many little ways inviolable patterns of daily life are established within the community group. *Individual privacy is restricted* by physical factors (large hospital wards, bedrooms (in residential homes) with several beds) and the need for fixed points in the individual's life emphasises the tendency to ritual and inflexibility. Block treatment—treating all those who live in the institution in the same way—reduces individuality and lowers self-esteem. This, too, emphasises the need for some personal possessions—the security of a personal chair, a private corner, etc.

A split between the resident group and the smaller staff group is based on the integration of the latter group into wider social systems and on the dependence of residents or patients on members of staff for physical and emotional care. A process of stereotyping takes place which includes feelings of hostility between both groups. From the staff point of view this involves feelings that residents are rejecting of help, and are often bitter and uncooperative. Patients and residents frequently feel guilty, anxious, afraid of the power of staff members, and vulnerable. One response to this split is *depersonalisation* which takes the form of denying recognition to the individuality, or wholeness, of the resident. Using first names, or calling older people 'Granny' or 'Pop', may be done to demonstrate affection or familiarity. Often it has a dehumanising effect: in failing to accord the privileges of name and title there is always a danger of reducing the person to an object. Many homes and hospitals can be seen to be full of clean, well-fed bodies but not of people.

Role-deprivation is a consequence of growing old: entry to an old people's home or hospital will involve role-loss. Those who go into an enclosed environment leave behind them many active roles; they may cease being tenants, householders or neighbours, they stop being people who pay the milkman or who hold their own rent book and collect their own pension. The loss of all these roles, and the reciprocal relationships that they imply at a time of other major life changes, adds up to considerable personal deprivation. It is vital that older people in institutions are given the opportunity to regain self-esteem and to rebuild their self-concept. One way of helping them to do this will be the simple recognition, by staff, of their right to respect and of their difference from other residents.

Ideally the social processes within the institutional organisation should and often do contribute to the therapeutic goals. It must be remembered, however, that the features of the total institution described by Goffman—the tendency for all residents to be treated alike, at the same time, in the same place—can lead to the unpleasant and anti-therapeutic features described above.

(ii) Institutionalisation: a concept of illness

Barton (1959) has described symptoms of an illness experienced by people living within institutions which he calls 'institutional neurosis'. This is caused by elements within the institution, particularly loss of contact with the outside world and complete submersion in the institutional system. Institutional neurosis may occur in all kinds of institutions—prisons, hospitals, monasteries and residential homes.

The patient or inmate becomes highly dependent as the personality is gradually eroded and apathy and withdrawal result. Typically the posture of the elderly patient shows the effects: slumped in a chair,

18

head bowed and with little facial expression, they take no interest in events happening around them. Older people seem particularly vulnerable to institutional neurosis which is associated with the negative elements of enclosed life which have already been described: ritualisation, rigidity, lack of privacy, stereotyping and role-deprivation. Whitehead (1970) suggests that three factors tend to perpetuate these conditions. He blames the lack of satisfactorily motivated staff, the fact that staff are often poorly trained and ignorant of the emotional needs of the elderly, and the problems of authoritarian hospital regimes which produce petty restrictions and staff fears.

In these kinds of circumstances it is hardly surprising that some older patients respond to pressure by sinking into withdrawal and deny the reality of their existence. An initial attempt to hide from the world becomes habitual and is made more rigid by the over-protection often found in nursing care of the elderly. The result is the institutional neurosis of Barton and is illustrated by several writers in descriptions of elderly people in a variety of circumstances.

(iii) What happens in enclosed residential communities providing care for the elderly?

There have been a number of very influential studies which highlight the way older patients and residents of old people's homes actually live and experience institutional care. A brief examination of three of the most significant of these will give some understanding of the positive and negative elements of long-term care.

In *The Last Refuge* (1962) Peter Townsend looked at the need for institutions and homes for old people and at the forms which they did take and also the forms which they should take. The book gives a brief history of residential care, describes the kinds of homes that exist for old people and the lives that residents lead. It also sets out to examine the reasons for old people giving up their own homes to live in residential care and gives some concluding recommendations on standards of care and future policy on provisions of long-term care. Townsend's study presented a picture of wide variations that led to very depressing conclusions. Homes showed gross inequalities, ranging from old workhouses with very little updating work done on them, through smaller buildings converted after the war (often with draughty corridors, steep stairs, bedrooms for five or six people, etc.), to very new small homes for from ten to twenty people, run by voluntary associations. In addition to the physical environment, the study showed up variations in treatment and attitudes in homes.

Although Townsend pointed to the advantages of regular meals, warmth, comfort, companionship and a degree of supervision and care he did also identify many disadvantages to residents. It was clear that most people in the homes would have been capable of living in appropriate housing in the community: physical infirmity was not too great to preclude this. Most people went into residential care because of a range of social factors: lack of money, lack of suitable housing, lack of adequate supportive help in everyday living. Entry into an old people's home for many of them meant loss of occupation and loss of contact with friends, family and the community in which they had been living. It meant also that they would experience difficulty in building relationships with either staff or other residents, that they would lose privacy, identity and powers of self-determination. Townsend recommended strongly, as a result of this study, that future policy should aim to make it possible for the elderly individual to continue to live an active, independent life in the community. It was important, he felt, to restore health, to provide continuing occupation, to facilitate the maintenance of family links and of a wide social support network which would enable individuality and independence to survive.

A few years later an association called Aid for the Elderly in Government Institutions (AEGIS) was formed and as a result of an appeal in *The Times* in November 1965 for information about the treatment of elderly hospital patients Barbara Robb produced *Sans Everything—A Case to Answer* (1967).

AEGIS was concerned particularly with older patients in the geriatric wards of general hospitals as well as those in mental hospitals where they did not belong. The book is a collection of letters from nurses and social workers, and of comments from professionals and observers. At the beginning of the campaign it was recognised that there were good hospitals, but members of AEGIS identified the very poor physical conditions—prison-like blocks, huge wards with few facilities, no baths, primitive toilets, bare walls and carpetless floors—which existed in some hospitals. Serious overcrowding and understaffing were identified as leading to inappropriate and unsuitable treatment of patients by staff and to irritability, frustration and degeneration among the patients.

The evidence and descriptions of six nurses, two social workers, and of Barbara Robb's own experience of attempting to rescue an elderly artist, Miss Wills, from a psycho-geriatric ward where she had been inappropriately abandoned, made a very convincing case for change in hospital environment and treatment. Several points were emphasised: the need for a comprehensive psycho-geriatric service; for the separation, from the mentally disturbed, of people who were in hospital because they were 'merely old'; for increased use of voluntary services in hospital; for encouraging visits from family and friends; and for having some personal possessions.

In his study *Taken for a Ride*, Meacher (1972) looked specifically at the treatment of confused elderly people in homes. He examined the assumptions underlying the tendency for many local authorities to establish special homes for confused elderly people. He suggested that it is widely regarded as undesirable to place confused older people in association with gross forms of mental illness and that special homes are seen as providing an environment in which the behaviour of confused residents will be less irritating to those around them. He agreed that confused actions can cause angry reactions but emphasised the importance of looking for positive counterbalancing factors in placing confused older people in ordinary residential homes.

He argued that although what he described as separatist homes for the elderly do offer advantages of administrative convenience, and they protect ordinary homes from repugnant behaviour, they do have negative aspects. Separatism may lead to stigmatisation in terms of resources, staff recruitment, etc., it may lead to very bizarre residential groups, it may conceal a system of control for difficult or aggressive elderly people, and it may lead to assumptions and stereotyping. An old person who is admitted to care, perhaps at a time of crisis, often with inadequate explanation or preparation, will be disturbed and may become disorientated. Once identified as confused they will be treated as a 'confused person' and without support and understanding may accept the role and continue to behave in a confused way.

Perhaps the most important suggestion of Meacher's study is that contentment and happiness among residents seem to be less likely to be achieved in separatist homes. He points to a link between the psycho-pathology of confusion and 'manifestations of insecurity, shallowness of relationships and unrequited affection'—manifestations which both Townsend and Robb identify as common in institutional care for the elderly.

All three books have made significant contributions to the development of institutional care for the elderly in generalised as well as specific ways. In the light of this discussion it begins to be possible to identify some of the meanings of the word institutionalisation in different contexts. In spite of the negative connotations which it has picked up, institutionalisation can be a useful concept. In a narrow, specific sense it can be taken to mean institutional neurosis in Barton's sense of illness manifestations. In a rather wider context it can refer to the organisational processes and the pressures that they put on individual people in institutional situations and which lead, in the extreme, to institutional neurosis, but in less extreme form to apathy, disinterest and withdrawal from active participation in relationships.

Aspects of communal living

The institution as an organisational system

It has already been suggested that each institution can be described as a social system in which a number of characteristic processes are carried out. Within the system are a number of different aims and goals. Miller and Gwynne (1972) have proposed two models of residential care which define the primary task of a residential institution in rather different ways. They suggest a warehousing model, in which the primary task is seen as the prolongation of human life, and a horticultural model, in which the primary task is seen as the development of the unsatisfied needs, drives, and unfulfilled capacities of the deprived individuals who live in care.

Although in many ways a helpful categorisation this does not take into account the fact that each member of staff and each resident, or patient, will have an individual view of the goals and tasks of the home or hospital. The way in which the formal organisation of the institution is constituted will relate to the overt objectives, the stated aims of the hospital, home, etc. The ways in which it actually functions and operates on a day-to-day basis will be more closely linked to the unspoken objectives of individuals—which may well vary from one moment to the next. Many studies of institutions have taken the view that they can be described and examined as self-contained units. Institutions do have fixed boundaries both physical and abstract but there are also many areas of interaction with the outside world. Processes of human interaction are in some aspects of institutional life very rigid and inflexible; in other aspects they are flexible and fluid.

It is possible to argue that problems arise out of structures within the institution—out of conditions which are inherent in the system such as allocation of financial control, therapeutic resources, etc., as much as out of decisions made within this set of conditions. One important element in overcoming these problems and promoting the effective fulfilment of institutional and individual goals is good communication. Poor or distorted communication may lead to conflict.

For the individual it seems likely that, as the Williams Report (1967) suggested, even the best residential home will rank as second best in the minds of those who come into it. Admission to an institution almost always involves the individual in loss, both of social roles and of material possessions. Additionally most admissions are the result of stressful situations in the community. Homelessness, family breakdown, illness, madness, parental rejection, crime, etc., are typical reasons for going into an institution.

The person going into a home, hospital or prison is commonly coming from a stressful situation and suffers the extra burden of facing up to the loss of what has gone before and the difficulties of joining a new group. He brings with him his own particular needs. He needs to influence and affect the other members of the new group, to impress upon them his own sense of identity. He needs, in other words, to preserve a sense of self. As well as this he brings the conflict between the need to feel secure, wanted and to be protected on the one hand and the need to remain a separate independent being on the other.

Institutions are made up of several elements: the aims of those involved (the aim of the community, the aims of the institution or the aims of the staff or residents, etc.), the organisational structure, and the residents and staff within the organisation. It has often been suggested that the conflict between those institutional goals which satisfy the needs of the resident and those which satisfy the needs of staff members is inevitable. The conflict may be drawn into the institution and become a conflict between the needs of staff members and those of the residents. There is some evidence (Teulings, Jansen and Verhoeven, 1973) that growth and scale enlargement of the hospital organisation is accompanied by qualitative changes in the social structure; that is, in the forms of division of labour and the distribution of power. It is suggested that there is no direct relationship between growth and development conditions and patient care (measured as a level of communicative behaviour on the part of the nurses) but there might be an indirect one. In the first instance the work-unit structure affects the quality of relationships and this in turn affects the nurse/patient relationship.

Menzies (1960) studied nurse/patient relationships and emphasised several elements in the social system which help to defend nurses against anxiety. She described the splitting up of the nurse/patient relationship, depersonalisation, detachment and denial, ritualisation rather than decision-making, passing upwards of responsibility, and an avoidance of change. Hanson (1971) looked at residential care for older people and identified four main problem areas. He describes 'block treatment' as putting the same demands on all residents irrespective of individual need and, growing out of this, 'regimentation'. He, too, emphasised 'depersonalisation', and also noted 'social distance' as the absence of conversation other than that which is staff initiated. The effect on the resident of these organisational pressures varies and apathy and withdrawal may be as much an angry reaction as violent behaviour or childishness.

Residential workers may sometimes fear involvement in inter-personal relationships with residents because of the anxieties that may be aroused by such involvement. One real problem is the inevitability of the breaking up of relationships following discharge, death or 'cure'. Less tangible are the anxieties aroused through relationships formed in enclosed situations: painful feelings that realistically belong to earlier relationships may become attached to very close relationships formed in circumstances of enforced physical or emotional dependence. Ritualisation and standardisation of task performance avoids the need for constant decision-making and the fear of making the wrong decision in these circumstances.

One way of looking at institutional behaviour is in terms of conflict relationships. A conflict relationship may be defined as a relationship in which the parties involved can gain relatively only at each other's expense. Conflict can arise because of 'position scarcity', meaning that a role cannot be simultaneously occupied by two people, or it can arise because of 'resource scarcity' when there is a limited supply of desired objects. Conflict may be functional: it stimulates interest and curiosity and it prevents stagnation. It is through conflict that problems can be aimed and solutions arrived at: conflict is the root of personal and social change. The institutionalisation of conflict leads to regularised procedures for change and for the handling of power. The perceived power of staff in institutions to give or withold desired objects (which may be taken to refer to objects giving either intrinsic or extrinsic satisfaction, or both) may lead to violence. Passive (structural) violence can be defined as that which creates a gap between what an individual needs (which demands a concept of human rights) and that which he is able to obtain. Active physical violence may be the extreme result of structural limitations placed on the individual.

In this sense regimentation, depersonalisation, role-deprivation, etc., can be seen as violent and as the expression of unrealistic conflict. It is because conflict becomes channelled through institutional structures that it loses its functional qualities and introduces destructive elements to the institution. These destructive elements are on at least two levels—on the level of the organisational structure, and in terms of the ways in which that structure impinges on those who have to live within it. Conflict within the organisational structure can be resolved in three main ways: it can be resolved by personalities within the organisation, or by building in additional organisational roles to cope with the existing conflict, or by altering the existing structure to remove conflict potential.

In arguing that violence, as defined here, is the result of institutionalised conflict I am arguing also for a total institutional strategy to reduce the danger of such violence. Conflict is inevitable, and can be functional. It is consequently important that conflict relationships are appropriately handled. I would suggest that one of the roles of a social worker within an institutional setting and of the residential worker is to participate in stimulating an institutional strategy that will enable conflict relationships to be realistically channelled. There seem to be two main areas of functioning that can be improved by such intervention.

Most importantly communication between individuals and groups can be improved. This will include communication between staff and staff, staff and residents, and residents and residents. The reduction of violence will follow improved communication and understanding which will create realistic conflict and therefore change. It is important, however, not to overestimate the power of communication: Etzioni (1960) suggests that the number of situations in which increased communication is likely to be effective is limited.

A second important area is the need for a range of substitute social experiences. It has been pointed out that admission to forms of care or containment involves role-loss. Through the creation of alternative role opportunities the resident can be offered a chance to maintain personal identity within an institution.

It is my suggestion, then, that physical violence in residential situations is an extreme form of the more common manifestations of passive violence. Both are created because of the unrealistic channelling of conflict and because of the pressure on individuals of the organisational structure. One important residential-work task is to become involved in the ways in which the institution impinges on the individuals within it. By improving communication, and offering alternative role opportunities, the worker can help to reduce the potential for violence.

Several Committees of Inquiry have drawn attention to the results that can occur if the potential for violence is not recognised and appropriately handled. One inquiry, for example, was instituted (Ely Report, 1969) following allegations in the *News of the World* in July 1967 by an ex-nursing assistant at Ely Hospital. He alleged cruel ill-treatment, inhuman and threatening behaviour towards patients, pilfering of food and clothing, indifference to complaints on the part of the chief male nurse and lack of care by the physician superintendent.

In concluding their report the members of the committee felt that the general situation had proved sufficiently disturbing to make the original concern justified. They reported undue roughness, and clumsiness during the course of handling patients (because of an acceptance of old-fashioned and unsophisticated techniques for controlling patients), unduly long periods of seclusion for one particular elderly patient, and another patient with a known capacity for impulsive violence was allowed to exercise too much authority. Food supplied for the patients was found to have been consumed by members of the ward staff but it was not established that pilfering extended to clothing. Recommendations were for the urgent relief of the overcrowding, an increase in staffing establishment, and corresponding efforts to recruit the necessary staff. In addition to this they felt there was a need for better training and improved status for nursing staff and better supervision. On a more general level there was a recommendation for close administrative co-operation within the NHS and a system of hospital inspection to prevent similar situations arising.

A further report concerning a home for about 270 adult males either mentally handicapped or severely mentally handicapped (Farleigh Report, 1971) again followed allegations that patients had been ill-treated by male nurses and the conviction of three nurses for a number of offences. Once again several points were highlighted: the difficulties of coping with violent patients, inadequate supervision, lack of training and guidance, overwork, overcrowding and the low status and morale of nursing staff. At about the same time the Secretary of State for Social Services in accepting the Whittingham Report (1972) said that the report revealed inadequate medical and nursing care for a large proportion of patients, misconceived and defective management policies and methods, and suppression of complaints from junior nurses. The committee also believed that there had been large-scale pilfering, if not more organised corruption on the part of some members of the staff.

Both passive and active overt violence clearly result when staff have little support, poor training and are under pressures of overwork and overcrowding as well as working in a low-status position.

Older people in care

Harris (1968) found that a high proportion of residents in old people's homes liked living in the home they were in. In one area the proportion of those saying they liked living in the home was as high as 90 per cent; in other areas it fell to between two-thirds and three-quarters of the residents. In only one area, with a high proportion of residents in older public assistance institutions, did the proportion of those liking the home fall as low as a half. Others said they liked the home they were in with some qualification. Only 12 per cent of residents were unhappy living in their home and this was mainly linked to having to share accommodation and to distance from family and friends. Harris had little doubt that most residents are quite content to be living in a home.

Slater (1968) studied the adjustment of forty residents to old people's homes using a measure of self-image and self-rating of health. He found that the length of stay, the level of physical disability, the number of friends made in the home, the number of visitors, and objection or acquiescence to denial of self-decision-making, all related to the level of adjustment of the residents as measured by their responses to his indexes. The more disabled residents had a better self-image (perhaps because they felt they received more specialised care for their needs) and the long-stay residents tended to be less positive about their 'life on the whole' than those who had been in only a short time.

Perhaps most important of all is the finding that social-relationship factors are very important in determining the level of adjustment:

Mr A was 87 years old when he was admitted to an old people's home. He had lived in a large Midlands town until the death of his wife three years earlier. For more than two years he remained alone in his rented flat with support from a home help and meals-on-wheels and a weekly visit from his only daughter who lived almost sixty miles away. She was herself almost at retirement age and her own children had left home.

Mr A's daughter eventually persuaded him to give up his flat and move to live in her large comfortable home: if her husband did not actually approve of this he seems to have raised no objections at the time. Mr A gave up the flat, gave away and sold most of his furniture and made the move.

It soon became apparent that he and his son-in-law were in competition for his daughter's care and attention. Each of the men took up a rigidly defended position and the daughter's position became unbearable. When Mr A and his son-in-law reached the point of physical violence the older man had to enter residential care.

Once there he continued to present as a rigid, defended personality who refused to recognise the existence of conflict at home: he insisted there was no reason for him to be in the residential home. He was unable to identify himself as an 'old person' and rejected contact with other residents, whom he saw as 'poor old folk'. He was continually in conflict with staff and residents over relatively minor matters such as mealtimes, bath-times, which window should be open or shut. He was, in other words, desperately anxious to be recognised as an individual. After his wife's death, his daughter's rejection, and finding himself far from his previous friends, he was lost, lonely and very frightened.

During this period he was asked to write down some of his feelings about old age and the home. He wrote as follows: 'I have been asked to write a few lines on the subject of growing old and living in an old people's home. As I am eighty-eight years of age and have spent nine months in a home I think I am in a position to do so. Of course some age quicker than others: I can only speak personally. Up to my middle seventies I didn't feel my age but I had gastric flue and it left me with a gastric stomach and interfered with my digestion. It did a lot to weaken me and now I am uncertain on my legs but I can't grumble as I haven't been troubled with rheumatism like a lot of old folk. Up to sixty years of age I never had any trouble but then I couldn't pass my water and had to go into hospital to be operated on for the removal of my prostate gland. Then I had shingles. Later I had a double hernia. I tire quickly now but that is the price to pay for living so long.

'I didn't like being in a home at first. It upset me to see so many people a lot more helpless than myself. This is a wonderful place and everything is done for them as humanly possible. I often marvel how the matron performs her numerous tasks. Some are so helpless—the inmates I mean—that they ought to be in hospital. And some, in my opinion, ought to be looked after by their families.'

Asked to commit himself to paper Mr A was unable to write about many of the things he had earlier articulated. Nevertheless the pain of his life is clear. He feels he cannot grumble about his health but his self-image is very closely linked to the physical changes and losses that ageing has brought: perhaps most of all ageing has brought threats to his masculinity. In describing the home he is apart from it, withdrawn into his own isolation. The residents to him are 'they', the 'inmates', poor old people with whom he cannot identify: perhaps the final comment is the most telling of all—'some, in my opinion, ought to be looked after by their families.'

Soon after this note was written another old man of similar age was admitted to the home for short-term care to give his family a rest. He eventually remained in the home and he and Mr A became good friends, always sitting together in a small lounge pulling their families and the other residents to pieces. Mr A began to become more settled in the home, talked rarely of moving to a flat outside and began to make more contacts in the home. The right kind of opportunity to interact with a suitable other person made a great deal of difference to his ability to adjust to his past losses and his current environment.

One other aspect of Mr A's comments is his ambivalent feelings towards the matron: regularly he felt angry and hostile towards her but felt he had to write about how marvellous she was. A similar pattern of ambivalence is, of course, evident in all dependency situations. In one hospital possibilities of extending group activities for elderly patients were explored and this raised problems of ambivalence in a number of ways:

A group of eight patients attended the first meeting, having been approached previously by the social worker: these patients were selected by nursing staff for their suggested intellectual ability to participate in discussion. They were told they were meeting to discuss whether they thought there was a need for a patients' committee and whether they wanted meetings of any other nature. A consistently non-directive approach to leadership was taken by the student and by the Occupational Therapist who ran the group jointly. In the first meeting patients were obviously very anxious at any suggestion that the patients should decide how to use the group, with staff members merely providing labour, several of them became quite agitated. One patient left the group during the first session and two others refused to come the following week.

Several points emerged clearly from this. The suggestion that patients might think and act for themselves within a group produced a definitely hostile reaction. This seems to be partly linked to confusion: the entire hospital regime is based on looking after patients at all times and this new message apparently conflicted with this; patients were consequently uncertain and frightened. It seems also to be partly connected with fantasies of staff power: it may be seen as unsafe to rebel against the existing pattern for fear of reprisals. A further element in the hostility that arose was the lack of a concrete group task: without an obvious purpose the patients found it hard to achieve any kind of group cohesion. Not only were the patients made anxious by the offer of independent thought but some members of staff found the group hard to understand. Difficulties about the patients meeting in the staff dining room were raised: problems about the group drinking tea from staff cups, and comments such as 'She may be all right with you but she always has diarrhoea when she comes back to the ward' were thrown out.

Institutional living—a summary

It should be plain from this discussion that living in an enclosed residential or hospital community means very different things to different individuals. Some general comments are possible, however; an institution is a social system within itself, in which there are no barriers between the activities of eating, sleeping, working and playing. The processes and structures within the institutional organisation may combine with factors affecting decision-making and communication to create situations in which passive and even active overt violence may result. The social worker in hospital, or the residential worker, has a role in clarifying communication and in interpreting the institution to the resident and patient and to offset some of the effects of institutional living. Residents who have the opportunity to build up social roles and relationships both inside and outside the institution are more likely to feel positive about their whole-life pattern. It is therefore important that residential workers should be able to facilitate a range of role choice.

Chapter three

Special needs of the elderly

Growing old is an increasingly common phenomenon: people live longer now than ever before and it is possible to look at some of the needs of all older people as a group. In addition to this it has to be accepted that minority groups of older people experience special problems which often combine and lead them to seek help from supporting services. These minority groups have needs which must be considered separately from general issues of 'old age'.

Rights of older people

In introducing a concept of rights I am not so much suggesting that some values are morally good, but rather proposing that particular values are necessary in an industrial society if older people are to lead their lives with basic opportunities for achieving satisfactions.

A reduction in the range of *choice* is commonly a result of living longer. As people grow older they begin to drop some of their social roles: this is more likely to happen to men than to women but is a factor in the life of all older people. The individual may be conceived of as the sum of the social roles that he plays; although this approach is very limited it is easy to see that a loss of roles involves a loss of reciprocal relationships and brings consequent loss of the satisfactions that attach to the relationships. The roles that are lost vary in significance from major roles involved in important social institutions such as employment and marriage, to lesser roles of shopper, or user of public transport. Retirement and widowhood bring loss of many relationships—workmate, canteen customer, employee, employer, husband, wife, etc. Along with this loss of roles and relationships goes the loss of many material opportunities—loss of income, decrease in mobility, etc. Each loss produces a consequent reduction of choice. This is particularly true of older people in hospital or residential care. Admission to institutional care emphasises loss: more roles have to be given up, relationships are cut off by geographical, transport, or financial considerations, and home and furniture may have to be given up.

The complexity and stereotyping of attitudes to old age and ageing has already been indicated. Hobman (1972) suggests that one solution to the difficulties that loss associated with ageing brings lies in the attitude of others surrounding ageing people. He feels that support from family, friends and neighbours in the community, given on the old people's terms, will enable them to continue to 'select and reject according to their own personal preferences and temperaments'. Choice should be a real possibility for older people. If they are to exercise choice then they must also know what is available to them. Information services have been inadequate, unsuitable and sometimes inaccessible: a comprehensive information service sufficiently flexible to be sensitive to individual requirements is essential.

Closely linked with the right of older people to continuing opportunities for choice in daily living is *the need for them to retain independence and individuality.* To be able to retain true independence they must be able to maintain an adequate income and a level of physical health and mobility. To achieve the latter involves meeting many subsidiary needs—adequate services to combat sight, hearing and dental deterioration, a proper nutritional standard, the maintenance of personal and household standards of cleanliness, proper care of the feet, and a good accessible health service. It is frequently suggested that old people treasure their independence and that every effort should be made to enable them to remain in their own houses, which is seen as synonymous with independence. Whilst I believe that most old people much prefer to be in their own homes I feel it is important to look carefully at the meaning of independence in this context. Each individual has a *right to appropriate accommodation* and at any one time this may be a private house, a sheltered-housing scheme, a hospital or an old people's home. A rigid insistence on remaining in the community may be counter-productive for a very small minority. In terms of the provision of accommodation it is again important to retain the element of flexibility and choice.

Beyond this it is important also not to confuse independence with the need for self-respect and dignity. In some senses many old people living very protected institutional lives, but able to dress themselves and move around in a wheelchair, may have a better self concept, and higher self-esteem—i.e. feel more independent—than others living in their own homes but only surviving with considerable physical support from others.

Linked with this concept of individuality is the right to *dignity and respect*. Stereotyped views of old age may lead to a tendency to an oversimplified perception and treatment of individuals. Treating people with respect involves looking beyond the stereotype to the whole needs of the individual. Older people have a right to be seen as individuals: in other words they have *a right to be different*. This is particularly important in an institutional context where intrusions into privacy are common, quiet corners are rare and the private world of the individual is vulnerable.

There should be no intrusion into privacy: respect for privacy is a part of the wider concept of respect for persons. The depersonalising effects of institutional living discussed in the previous chapter should be prevented. Some older people, of course, are well able to take care of themselves:

Mr B was 67 years of age and totally blind when he was admitted to an old people's home. He had lived alternately with his daughter and his sister after the death of his wife some years before and when, following his daughter's illness, his sister began to find her own sight failing he was admitted to care, ostensibly as a short-term measure.

In the home, he found himself to be at least ten years younger than most of the residents and felt separated from them by his blindness. He rapidly became bored and apathetic and spent much of his time in his own room smoking and stubbing out his cigarettes in the washbasin. The officer in charge of the home objected to both the smoking in the bedroom ('because he's blind') and the method of his disposal of the ash. Her attitude proved the saving of Mr B: he took up the challenge and continued his smoking and extended his activities to disappearing for long walks alone and causing considerable worry!

In prolonging the fight he was able to rebuild his feeling of identity after his family's rejections (as he perceived it) and he preserved his individuality through a cheerful conflict. The staff were able to recognise this and accept him within the communal group.

Satisfaction and happiness

These fundamental rights to choice, respect, dignity, independence, individuality and privacy are relevant only in so far as they provide for satisfaction in old age. Satisfaction depends also on external, material factors as well as on the internal dispositions of the ageing person. It has already been suggested that ambivalence is one element of the response to ageing. Margery Fry (1954, p. 8), at the age of 80, suggested some of the dilemma:

> The ebb and flow of strength must be learned and accepted by those who suffer it... the sense of uselessness weighs heavy on many old people, particularly on those who have put themselves eagerly into their work, and above all, those whose work has been largely in helping others, such as mothers of families. It may almost be described as the penalty for a life well spent.

Personal satisfaction seems to be a fundamental need: to be able to feel that life is purposeful and meaningful is vital. Erikson (1950) has proposed that the process of growing from childhood through adulthood to old age requires the successful negotiation of a series of identity crises leading to a final stage of ego integrity. The achievement of ego integrity involves an acceptance of past life—of all that has gone before—as inevitable and unchangeable, a recognition that the present is meaningful in the light of what has happened in that past life, and a realisation that death is an unavoidable and appropriate conclusion.

In this sense satisfaction in old age is dependent on being able to see a total pattern in life. This will not be easy for some people; some may feel that their life has been unproductive, or that their present circumstances are not a just reward for a lifetime of hard work. The deprivations that many older people suffer are often the result of the unpredictable failure of health or of the external effects of actions taken by the wider society. It is therefore not enough to see the achievement of inner satisfaction as solely a matter for the internal adjustment of the individual. Satisfaction and happiness (which are not necessarily the same but are interconnected) depend on the congruence of the inner mental state with external circumstances.

'Normal' ageing processes

Ageing, it is often suggested, is a process in which we are all involved to a greater or lesser extent. Chronological events during this process cannot effectively be related to normality in the current state of knowledge but only to statistical and numerical frequency. Ageing involves the continual interaction of a great many variables, physical, social, intellectual and emotional and it is difficult to identify what is natural or normal during ageing because of the range of variables. It is perhaps easier to identify what is 'common' or usual, but that can sometimes be misleading (Hall, 1972).

The concept of ageing as a process implies that the individual has to negotiate a series of transitional phases of life during his progress through a life-cycle or in negotiating what Bromley (1974) has called the life path. To pass successfully out of one of these stages of development or ageing is to pass into a new phase of life. The main implication of this is that growing old involves continually progressing to something new. It tends to play down, while not completely precluding, the fact that some parts of the life process involve a degree of marking time, without significant change either social, physiological or emotional.

One value of being able to view ageing as an ongoing process is that it points the way to appropriate solutions that must be provided by caring services. The problems of older people are often the result of blocks to important life goals. The removal of these blocks will allow the normal process of ageing to proceed: solutions are only relevant in so far as they relate to the restoration of this process.

A social process

A good deal of thinking about ageing as a social process has centred on the disengagement process. Broadly, it has been postulated (originally by Cumming and Henry, 1961) that social ageing involves the withdrawal of social supports and involvement from the older person; at the same time the older person accepts, and needs, this withdrawal. The picture of the disengaged older person is that of someone with very few social contacts, with few significant (in the sense of producing changes in behaviour) relationships, and with a reduction in ego energy available to seek out and use relationships. One disadvantage of accepting disengagement theory as a basis for providing helping services is that it would lead logically to providing little support or social contact for older people, and a decreasing amount of involvement as people become very old. There is ample evidence that decreased social stimulation can lead to loss of satisfactions for many older people and certainly the very old are making increasing demands on the caring services.

Discussion of disengagement has taken many forms and another approach has been that of Havighurst (1968) who has argued that happiness and satisfaction are within the reach of the great majority of people but many people are demonstrably unhappy and dissatisfied. He argues that there are some people who are relatively high in role-activity but would like to be more disengaged yet there is also evidence that for some people as the level of activity decreases so also do the individual's feelings of contentment. As Bromley (1974) has pointed out, the disposition to disengage is a personality dimension as well as a characteristic of ageing.

As people grow old they are certainly likely to disengage in the sense of losing roles. Some of the nature of role-loss has already been described. Blau (1973) suggests that the concept of role-loss, which is so commonly used, tends to emphasise the involuntary character of role-loss, and especially of retirement and widowhood. Events such as graduation or marriage do not have the negative connotations associated with retirement or widowhood, perhaps because the former two imply not just a departure from one status but an entry into another status. Blau believes that 'role-exit' is a more suitable description for the effects of ageing on roles because it is a more neutral and more comprehensive term. She feels that role-exit has three specific effects on the individual: 'it produces changes in an individual's associational life, his self-concept and his mood', the nature of these effects being to some extent dependent on the availability of alternative roles and relationships.

A cross-national study of old people in three industrialised societies (Shanas et al., 1968) looked at the problems of role, role-change, and disengagement. The authors concluded that older people as a whole are fairly well integrated into society by the kinds of services they receive from children, friends and neighbours and the services that they give in return. They are quite effectively knitted into the community groups within which they live by the reciprocity and interaction of the relationships that they have. The authors of the study did, however, go on to say that although most older people are well integrated there is a considerable minority segregated which are often associated with ageing.

The pattern of these social processes that emerges, then, is one of gradual lessening of involvement for most old people who tend to play fewer active roles in the wider society but who perhaps tend to get more intensive satisfactions from the fewer roles that remain to them. Certainly old people as a group do remain integrated into society and continue to achieve satisfaction from participation in relationships. For a few older people rather more roles may be lost for a number of reasons: some may choose to withdraw and actually enjoy disengagement, some may experience a crisis, such as sudden illness, bereavement, etc., and be unable to recover from the blow. It is this group of people—who are compulsorily disengaged from roles and relationships but who wish to remain engaged—who are most likely to require help and at worst admission to institutional care.

A physical process

The ageing organism is altered by the effects of heredity, environment and disease factors which produce characteristic common changes seen in the elderly. The rate at which these changes occur is by no means uniform and they are affected by the internal dispositions of the individual as much as by external environment. Some people survive by fighting and thrive on struggle and hard work but often age at no faster or slower a rate than others who live a protected and dependent existence. Some particular changes can, however, be highlighted.

Many older people undergo postural changes, and progressive decline in stature is usual: the elderly are characterised by shortened trunks and comparatively long extremities—in fact the reverse proportions to those seen in infancy. Height is lost partly as a result of changes in the intervertebral discs but also because of an increased attitude of flexion; flexion at the knees and at the hips tends to contribute further to diminishing stature. Facial changes, especially wrinkling, take place. The creasing of the skin due to the repeated use of the muscles of expression leads eventually to wrinkling, and habitual patterns of expression are formed. The loss and redistribution of subcutaneous fat contributes to and accentuates this wrinkling. Loss of fat from around the eyes leads to the typically sunken appearance of the eyes of elderly people. The loss of fat and elastic fibres leads to a laxness of the skin and in some people sagging of the tissues of the neck may produce a double chin. The development of *arcus senilis*, a white line encircling the cornea, is sometimes cited as evidence of ageing but is perhaps given over-emphasis. Greying of the hair tends to precede loss of hair: follicles become fewer and body hair and pubic and axillary hair begins to be lost. None of these changes, of itself, is evidence of ageing but their existence together contributes to building up the picture of a typical older person.

Other important changes should be mentioned. In the eye presbyopia, a form of longsightedness, develops from the 40s onwards involving a gradual reduction of the visual fields, a higher threshold for light stimulation, and a slowing of dark adaption (Agate, 1970). The ear begins to show changes at about the same age (around 45 years), with a gradually increasing threshold for higher frequencies. Characteristically, older people tend to develop a gradually increasing high-tone hearing loss and they sometimes have difficulty in picking out conversation between several people, or more non-specific conversation. There are many other basic organic changes which may be inherent in the structure of the organism. The ageing person manifests an increasingly limited capacity to respond to stress and the likelihood of death is increased because the longer a person lives the more likely he is to acquire a collection of illness and disease. If age-changes can be modified then the organism is better able to cope with physical stress and life is more likely to be prolonged.

Special needs of the elderly

An intellectual and emotional process

Most people as they grow older remain the same kind of person that they have been—only more so: there is a tendency for basic personality traits to become rather more entrenched and exaggerated. Some characteristic age-related changes in intellectual performance have been suggested.

The peak of creative ability seems to be reached comparatively early in life. Wechsler (1939, 1958) measured adult intelligence on the basis of performance on tests of intellectual ability (vocabulary, comprehension, etc.). The tests involved the ability to reason from one series of operations to another and were called 'don't hold' tests. The ability to perform 'hold' tests—involving the ability to reproduce well-learned information—remains constant throughout adult life but the ability to perform 'don't hold' tests shows a gradual decline with ageing. There is, in other words, a difference between reasoning and wisdom (Chown, 1972b). As people grow older they are more likely to accumulate knowledge as they solve new problems but the older they become the less likely they are to meet new problems.

Since older people are slower at doing most things than younger people it might be thought that this could account for some of the decline in performance. In fact Chown and Davies (1972) found older and younger people spent proportionately similar amounts of time on solving easy or difficult problems but that older people persisted longer on 'easy items' and gave up more quickly on 'difficult items'. The suggestion is that older people may require more cues than younger ones before they have an adequate basis for their judgments and will therefore have to process more information before reaching a conclusion. The consequence of this is that decision-making tends to take rather longer and older people are also more cautious, especially in giving advice. Memory loss is also common: although older people are able to learn they tend to require more time, depending on the nature and familiarity of the task. Short-term memory loss is one important element in the ability to solve problems and retain learning: short-term memory seems less efficient in older than younger people. Performance is, of course, very much dependent on motivation, interest, concentration, etc.

Older people tend to be pessimistic rather than optimistic. They are likely to see the world as a more hostile, less loving place and they are less likely to give emotional responses. There is sometimes said to be a cooling off, or flattening, of emotions. In addition to this older people may show a narrowing of interest, an increasing interest in the self, and some preoccupation with bodily functions: older people score higher on scales for hypochondriasis and hysteria. It is

sometimes claimed that increasing rigidity of thought is a characteristic ageing trend but Chown (1972a) suggests that most age-
related data concerning rigidity of thought are better looked at as
intelligence-related data.

It cannot be too often emphasised that ageing is a highly
individual process and each person follows a unique life-course that
depends on who he has been and what he has lived through. The
emotional life of most people develops and continues to take place
within a family group. It is the family that provides a safe base from
which to view and approach the world and within his family the
individual preserves and develops his self-image—his identity and
integrity. As the family develops it can be described in terms of a
total life-cycle in which the younger and older members are perform-
ing tasks at opposite ends of an unbroken continuum. In this view
the family life-cycle is a continuous spiral—although it may also be
seen as a series of parallel cycles or spirals followed by each of the
group of people who make up the family.

Certain tasks are more appropriate to particular age-ranges in the
family's development. The early part of the development is concerned with a stage of intimacy in which husband and wife learn to
be together, dependent on each other yet separate adults. As they
grow in knowledge of each other they move into a stage of child-
bearing and child-rearing. This begins a period which is concerned
largely with functions of caring—caring for children and perhaps
also caring for ageing parents. During this period, as people move
into middle age, they begin to achieve a high degree of security and,
outwardly, behaviour is stable and regular. It is a time for con-
solidation of earlier achievements from the vantage point of security
and safe routine.

Blenkner (1965) proposed that one important task of middle age
was the achievement of filial maturity. She suggests that as a person
reaches middle age he is forced to perceive his parents as no longer
entirely dependable and in some cases as dependent on him. This
requires a readjustment of attitude, which Blenkner calls the filial
crisis: the successful negotiation of this crisis leads to 'filial maturity'.
It is certain that ageing families experience changes in the patterns
of dependence within the group and adjustments have to be made.
Growing up through adolescence involves coming to terms with
being an independent, whole person who can yet retain relationships
with significant others. Growing old involves the reverse process—
coming to terms with increasing physical dependence yet remaining
a self-respecting person.

Arguably dependence is an inevitable element of all relationships:
one side of a relationship involves dependence and the other involves
being depended upon. These elements are fluid and the balance

changes from one situation to another. One important task of the ageing individual is to learn to accept increasing dependence in a way that will still permit him to function as an independent individual. The pressures of loss associated with ageing can usually be coped with gradually but this is particularly difficult if losses are sudden and unexpected. The ways in which losses are handled will depend heavily on the way in which the individual perceives himself and his long-term expectations, and on the degree of motivation. Coping mechanisms are learned and carried out on the basis of these kinds of internal dispositions but are also dependent on external environments and supports.

Responses to stress at any age show tendencies to become preoccupied with the immediate future and with self-protection. Stress in old age will be handled as it would be handled at any age but some mechanisms may be more common. Older people seem to be more likely to project inner uncertainties and frustrations on to the outside world: this is reflected in the tendency to see the world in less loving terms that has already been discussed. They may also be more likely to regress to earlier patterns of behaviour: some nutritional feeding problems and some element of incontinence can be seen in the light of regressive defences. It is important not to confuse regression with the habit of reminiscing—which may represent realistic attempts to discover positive coping mechanisms in the past.

Frustration may be turned inwards and take the form of depression, or unhappiness, or it may be turned outwards as aggression and hostility. It is often those who provide most care for older people who are the most vulnerable to this displaced hostility. A normal ageing process must include opportunities to achieve a satisfying emotional equilibrium, involving a balance between inner needs and drives and external environment.

Individual aspects of ageing

It has already been suggested that many older people do remain closely involved in relationships and social activities. Some older people, however, experience problems which are not necessarily caused by ageing but are age-related. Most people are able to cope with the barriers to a satisfying process of life with the help of family and friends but a minority require help from caring services.

Occupational changes

Retirement is usual in our society: most men retire at the age of 65 and most women at the age of 60. The actual response to retirement, and expectations of the retirement period, tend to vary according to occupational and economic groupings. Some studies in the USA (Kerckhoff, 1964; Streib and Schneider, 1971) have found differences in attitude to retirement according to occupational class. Those in white-collar occupations tended to look forward to retirement but found it somewhat disappointing, those in professional occupations didn't welcome it but were able to enjoy it, and those in blue-collar occupations were fairly non-committal before the event but were less satisfied after retirement. Crawford (1972) in a British study found four main groupings of attitude to retirement. One group of men, largely in non-manual employment, saw retirement as a time to enjoy freedom and leisure and looked forward to giving up work. A second group of men, mainly in manual jobs, found most of their satisfactions in relationships at work and in work-related roles and feared retirement. A group of women, mainly the wives of non-manual workers, found satisfactions in their home and family and saw their husband's retirement as an opportunity to extend this. The final group tended to be the wives of manual workers who dreaded their husbands' retirement because it would limit their own activities outside the home.

There seems to be some relationship between adequate income and good health and enjoyment of retirement. Enjoyment of leisure requires sufficiently good health and perhaps enough money to engage in a range of activities. In Britain men tend to see the retirement period, in general terms, as a time when they can sit back and rest after a lifetime of labouring, in contrast to the USA where it is seen as the time to enjoy all the things that couldn't be done before.

Leisure is an important part of life and the opportunity for play is necessary at all ages: play is one vital element in a child's development and remains an essential part of self-expression in old age. Unfortunately many older people, having lived through two world wars and a series of economic crises, have often not had the chance to learn how to use leisure. Adult educational facilities should be geared to linking leisure and occupational interests to enable people to learn to play. Adult education has the additional, important, role of supplying companionship and social contacts for some older people.

Whatever the expectation of retirement the reality for most people brings economic change. Many older people are reliant on retirement pensions and on Supplementary Benefits and this has implications for the use made of leisure. Some older people do continue to work, and any retired person is eligible to register for employment with the local labour exchange. Voluntary and independent employment bureaux are also offering help to retired workers but with mixed success. Additional pressures exist to discourage or hinder attempts to find work after retirement: married women for instance, are more likely to take part-time jobs and compete with retired workers. The earnings rule, which puts a limit to the amount that can be earned before the pension is reduced, has also been a disincentive.

Retirement brings significant life changes. It brings loss of roles associated with work, and loss of family status as breadwinner. It also puts new demands on family communication patterns and it brings new economic pressures to the family. For many people retirement will create feelings of anxiety and stress and, for some, feelings of depression and unhappiness. It is therefore important to consider issues of retirement preparation. Many pre-retirement courses are run currently on the basis of perhaps half a dozen lectures on health and finance, held a few months before retirement. Although these may be a help to some, the significant issues of retirement, especially economic preparation and learning to use leisure, can most effectively be considered earlier in life. A change in wider attitudes to old age and retirement is necessary if the retirement period is to be effectively enjoyed by the majority.

One special recent trend in retirement has been the move to seaside resorts. Karn (1977) suggests that people do this for a number of reasons—a supposedly better climate by the sea, ill-health, to get away from towns to quieter places, housing needs, wishing to join friends or relatives, and to seek a complete change. This trend has created unbalanced populations in the retirement areas with consequent problems. There is an increased pressure on the social and health services but fewer younger people to meet the demand and often less money available because incomes tend to be seasonal and, on average, lower in resorts. Additional problems result as retired couples grow older and more infirm but have few local contacts on which to rely for support, especially when one partner dies.

Accommodation changes

The three major items of expenditure for old people—and for all of us—are food, housing and heating (Age Concern, 1971). Older people are likely to have to spend proportionately more of their income on housing than does the community as a whole. Poverty can be taken to refer not just to lack of income but also to deprivation of suitable environmental and material provisions. Housing that may have been adequate sixty years previously may have deteriorated to an unacceptable level or it may be that increasing infirmity makes the older person unable to use his house fully—bathroom and bedroom may be inaccessible up steep stairs. Inadequate accommodation, or the anticipation of increasingly inadequate housing is one of the commonest reasons behind applications for admission to residential care for the elderly. More sheltered housing schemes may help to reduce this problem.

Loneliness

Loneliness is hard to define but it is a feeling that is subjectively experienced by a fairly large minority of older people. Loneliness can be defined as a wish for contact with other people which cannot be achieved. It is an unpleasant internal disposition, related to unhappiness, which may be experienced in a communal situation as well as in isolation. Old people are eight times more likely to live alone than are people aged under 65 (Tunstall, 1966) but very old people are rather less likely to be on their own than the newly retired (Ministry of Pensions and National Insurance, 1966). Tunstall found a link between loneliness and isolation: those who are more isolated in the sense of having fewer contacts are more likely to say they are lonely.

It is possible to draw a distinction (Shanas et al., 1968) between peer-contrasted isolation, or having few social activities and relationships in comparison with age-contemporaries, and desolation. Desolation is used to refer to being deprived of formerly significant relationships and activities, often through death. Isolation tends to be related to being older than average, single or widowed, without children or relatives living nearby, retired or infirm. Perhaps the most important point about loneliness and social loss is that there seems to be a positive response to substitute relationships. In a long-stay setting loneliness is a feeling that may subjectively be described and may be related not so much to lack of contacts as to social loss or deprivation. One of the tasks of the worker in the long-stay situation will be to help the older person adjust to the loss and learn to make use of the available substitutes.

Family and friendship changes

On the whole older people do maintain friendships. A study in Nebraska (Booth and Hess, 1974) found that, of a sample of 800 older people, respondents claimed on average 4·2 people described as 'closest friends'. Married women were more likely to report friends of the opposite sex than widowed or single women. A comparison of the age-groups 45—64 and over 65 found no significant differences in the pattern of friendships for married and unmarried men, but significant differences across all categories of friendships for women. This seems to be linked to the increased mortality rate for men which means there are fewer men to go around. Married couples can maintain friendships but very often a widowed man or woman finds it hard to continue old friendships after bereavement.

As parents grow older the extent of their contact with children increases (Shanas et al., 1968). Families do usually accept a responsibility to care for their ageing members and will sometimes be reluctant to surrender that responsibility to social or health services. In a few cases this results in a crisis of family breakdown when the burden cannot be carried any longer: if this does happen it may leave a residue of guilt and anxiety after the crisis.

Some aspects of dependence in the family have already been discussed: the caring role of children becomes more important, often as the grandchildren are growing through adolescence and presenting families with separate anxieties. These elements of dependence are commonly contained within the family but in some cases may be channelled into neurotic satisfactions. The older person may use his dependence in a demanding way to gain power or control, much as a demanding baby can rule the household. Conversely children may take delight in punishing vulnerable, elderly parents for early-life conflicts.

As more people live longer so it becomes more likely that marriage partnerships are extended. There are more years together after the children leave home and these may be enjoyed, tolerated, or become unbearable: a marriage that has barely survived 'for the sake of the children' may be impossible with enforced companionship after retirement. There is no reason why sexual relationships should not continue into late life: habit seems to be a very important element in this.

There is no doubt that single and childless people are more vulnerable in later years, perhaps mainly because of the lack of support from families.

Bereavement, death and dying

It might be argued that as people age they have an expectation that those around them will die and, being better prepared than younger people, should be less distressed. Whether this is true or not, growing old involves having to perceive the reality of one's own death and making individual adjustments. To some extent this may be a task of middle age rather than of old age. Younger people may hide from seeing death in a personal sense and view it in secondary terms as something that happens to other people, but middle age presents physical changes which highlight the approach of death which has to be seen in personal terms. Making adjustments to this is therefore a task which many older people have already begun to work through. Fear of death is often associated with fear not of death itself but of the pain which goes with death, or is expected to go with death.

Loss of all kinds is associated with a subsequent period of adjustment or grieving. Grief is not only linked with loss of a person but can also relate to loss of a part of the self, or of good health, or of a house or possessions. It is to be expected, then, that older people entering a home or hospital will require a period of grieving which may take several forms. It is possible to describe common elements of the grieving process. In the first few days a feeling of emptiness, numbness and disbelief is common in which denial is a common feature. After this a period of grief, despair and emptiness follows in which episodes of physical distress alternate with apathy and disinterest. Sometimes anger, relief or guilt are felt. Appropriate grieving will normally require outlets of expression: if these are not available pathological reactions—chronic grief—may occur with excessive guilt, bitterness, anger or anxiety in evidence and occasionally hallucinations, delusions and physical reactions.

Dying, as such, is not a problem: it is a logical and inevitable conclusion to the ageing process. The pain or distress that may go with dying can create problems and difficulties for the dying person and his family. Most people who die are old, but men tend to die at an earlier age. The majority of people die in hospital or other institutions (Cartwright et al., 1973) but it is doubtful whether the staff are equipped to deal with dying people: education in the caring professions has tended to neglect this area of care. It is important that staff think carefully about how they will use the knowledge that a patient is dying and how they will treat him. They must be clear about their own fear of death and not allow it to become mixed up with their perception of the patient's fear. Hospitals should put more emphasis on caring and relieving rather than curing and treating if dying patients are to achieve what has been called a 'joyful process of dying' (Lamerton, 1973). Of course physical and emotional pain does exist but this can be minimised by medical care, and a recognition of the emotional needs of dying people can help to reduce their anxiety and fear.

Illness and disability

Older people tend to come to their GP for treatment fairly late in the evolution of disease (Williamson et al., 1964) and so studies of the incidence of disease have been hindered. Late reporting, or failure to report illness, has several causes: the slow onset of disease with minimal symptoms can only be detected by careful screening. Some older people deny the existence of symptoms and fail to go to the doctor because of their anxieties. Others confuse disease processes with stereotypes of elements of the ageing process, feeling that they are not ill, only growing old. Studies have found as much as 75 per cent of samples with at least one unknown moderate or severe disability (Williamson et al., 1964; Williams et al., 1972), and a similar proportion with significant unknown diseases.

It has often been proposed that an important prerequisite for the optimum deployment of medical and welfare services is the establishment of an at-risk register of elderly living at home (Gilmore and Caird, 1972). Some categories of older people are demonstrably at greater risk than others (Meacher, 1970): the severely incapacitated, the mentally infirm, those in extreme social isolation, those over 85, the recently bereaved and those with lesser chronic incapacity. A study by Gilmore (1975) of 300 old people in their own houses in Glasgow found that factors relating to mortality were the presence of arteriosclerotic disease, central nervous systemic disease, organic brain syndrome and other psychiatric disorders, limited mobility, physical disability, cigarette-smoking, poor recent memory and poor calculation ability. The range of illness and disability is very wide: a high degree of deficiency, disability and disease exists within the elderly population. Although many of these changes are taken for granted by the elderly and are not reported, a significant proportion is open to relief or removal (Skelton, 1972).

The physical changes which are commonly associated with the ageing process, as well as the accumulation of disease and disability, combine to bring about changes in self-image. We each have a view of ourselves which includes expectations of physical capacities. For some people physical factors—strength, beauty, etc.—are more important than for others and age-related changes make a re-appraisal of the self concept inevitable and this may bring associated problems. It will be difficult after fifty years in the same house not to be able to use the bath, to do the garden, clean the windows, or climb the stairs and to have to adjust not only to being unable to cope with these tasks but also to having to rely on others for help. Physical change may lead to increased dependency on others, to frustration, and depression or irritability. It will also emphasise the approach of death as a real, personal event.

Two particularly important aspects of physical change are incontinence and nutritional needs. Incontinence is important not only because of the distress it causes older people and those who care for them, but also because of the difficulties it creates in hospital and residential care and in transfering from the former to the latter. Incontinence can be defined as passing urine or faeces at unsuitable times or in unsuitable places (Agate, 1972). Most people who are incontinent can either be treated medically or can be encouraged and helped to manage their problems by habit-training, improving accessibility of toilets, etc. Some older people are incontinent because of anxiety, depression or apathy; others regress and behave in a childlike way, using incontinence to express aggression or hostility, or to further their dependence. The emotional element in incontinence can be an important one and treating the underlying unhappiness may help to build up self-respect and self-esteem and therefore encourage continence.

Similar emotional and psychological considerations might also be applied to nutritional and feeding behaviour in the elderly. There are, of course, realistic difficulties in maintaining a balanced, healthy diet: difficulties in reaching shops, in low incomes, lack of information and education, combine and may lead to insufficient food being consumed, or to obesity. In addition to these practical elements, over-eating or food refusal in the elderly can be seen as an expression of unhappiness, and treatment should be aimed at the underlying dissatisfactions.

Older people, then, are likely to accumulate disease and disability: often they display a multiplicity of illnesses and about two-thirds to three-quarters of the elderly at home have unreported disease or disability of a significant nature. It is important to remember, in providing long-term care for the elderly, that physical changes bring emotional and psychological changes which must be recognised and appropriately handled by those who provide care.

Psychiatric changes

Studies of mental illness in the community have shown that between 41 per cent and 55 per cent of elderly people living in their own homes have some psychiatric disorder (Whitehead, 1974). In addition to this almost half the patients in psychiatric hospitals are over 65. Diagnosis and classification of mental disorders in old age is complicated because of the brain changes which are commonly associated with ageing. Some classification may be attempted under the following headings: (1) acute brain failure, (2) chronic brain failure, (3) affective disorders. Most classifications also include late paraphrenia as a separate grouping. Brain failure, or brain syndrome, is a term that is preferred to senile dementia because it relates to a physiological or clinical state rather than to a complete disease process, involving aetiology, pathology, etc.

(1) Acute brain failure
Other terms used to describe this state are acute brain syndrome,

toxic confusional state, and acute delirium. The onset is characteristically unexpected, not so much in the sense of being sudden or dramatic, but in relation to a specific incident. The old person becomes bemused, lost, disorientated, may wander or become incontinent, and there is usually a fluctuating disturbance in the level of consciousness. Sometimes he is deluded or hallucinating. The most common precipitant of acute brain failure is infection but it may also be related to neurological, cardio-respiratory, endocrine or nutritional changes. Almost any disease can cause a state of confusion in older people but it may also be linked to other factors such as trauma, anaesthetic agents or sudden isolation.

(2) Chronic brain failure

There are many causes of brain damage, some of which may be reversible, while others may be irreversible or progressive. The main varieties of organic brain failure are cerebral arteriosclerosis and senile cerebral disease, although these two are not mutually exclusive.

The arteriosclerotic type of brain syndrome usually begins in late maturity and is characterised by failing memory, emotional liability, and wandering. Headaches, giddiness and blackouts may occur, short-term memory impairment increases and concentration deteriorates. Central personality traits may be preserved for some time; the more subtle features of personality suffer. The onset often follows a cerebral vascular accident and it is associated with changes in the circulation of blood to the brain. In contrast the onset of senile psychosis, or senile dementia, is rather more gradual: intellectual deterioration is slow but progressive. It is characterised by memory impairment, blunting of the emotions, loss of interest, irritability and restlessness. It is distinguished from normal ageing mainly by the extent and rigidity of changes. Eventually social and emotional behaviour loses all coherence and the speech and thought disintegrate.

Other chronic organic brain changes take place and some presenile dementias have been defined. Alzheimer's disease seems to be due to a primary degenerative process almost identical to that found in many cases of senile dementia. Emotional disturbances occur with attacks of depression or euphoria; self-neglect and purposelessness are common and muscle rigidity occurs in the latest stages. Pick's disease begins with a slow deterioration in behaviour, with blunting of the emotions and childish behaviour. Other, less common, pre-senile dementias are Jakob-Creutzfeldts disease, and Huntingdon's Chorea, and chronic brain failure may also be associated with syphilis, alcoholism, trauma and tumour.

(3) Affective disorders

There is an expectation that older people will be slower in their thoughts and actions, will have difficulties with sleeping and concentration, and will be more self-centred, showing less interest in the outside world. These and other factors complicate the diagnosis of depression in the elderly. This is further complicated by the presentation of a similar picture to that of dementia (Whitehead, 1974). Depression may be a normal or natural outcome of bereavement, or any of the losses that older people are likely to experience, or it may be endogenous—from within the old person with no immediately obvious cause. The depressed person cries frequently, may feel guilty or anxious, becomes preoccupied with health and bodily functions, and complains of sleeping difficulties. Although usually well orientated, in advanced cases depression leads to apathy and withdrawn negativism which may easily be mistaken for dementia. Other disorders of the emotions are mania and hypomania, which are not common in the elderly but which do occur. The manic is over-active and excited, often sleeps badly and has a poor appetite. There is a feeling of well-being but no insight and the danger of the associated over-activity is the exhaustion that may result in older people.

(4) Late paraphrenia

This condition is sometimes described as 'schizophrenia of late onset' and it is characterised by paranoid, aggressive actions and delusions, but also by shrewd intelligent behaviour in some sections of functioning. The principal difficulty of the condition is that older people who suffer from it tend to shut themselves away, rejecting help and making accusations at those around them.

The important difference, from the point of view of providing care, between physical change and psychiatric change is that the former requires attitudinal changes mainly in the ageing person while the latter requires attitudinal adjustments on the part of caring relatives, friends and neighbours. It is not easy to tolerate an old person who wanders at night, or who develops unsociable habits. There is a danger, in extreme circumstances, of families falling into the habit of seeing confused behaviour as done on purpose, or out of spite. It is also difficult to care for older people who make accusations of theft, etc., perhaps because of paranoid ideas but also because of unsuccessful attempts to put a disordered world back into order. Putting money away for safe-keeping, they may forget where the money is and accuse the home help of stealing it. Mental disorder is hard to deal with in any situation and requires particularly careful thought in communal groups.

Needs of the elderly — a summary

In reviewing the kinds of needs that older people bring to hospital or to residential care it is possible to look at general needs of older people as a group, as well as at the specific needs of individual patients or residents. As a group older people have a right to live satisfying lives and in order to do that they should be able to exercise choice within a flexible environment to achieve a balance between inner needs and external pressures. In addition to this some other criteria of adequate adjustment can be suggested: it is important to be able to see a continuity between past, present and future, and to be able to accept the inevitability and 'rightness' of death. Perhaps most importantly older people need financial and material security in order to be able to achieve emotional security. Individuals entering institutional care do so because they have come up against barriers to the normal ageing processes which lead to satisfaction. The objectives of long-term care should be aimed at the restoration of those processes and at facilitating the achievement of individual satisfactions.

Chapter four

Entering care

Admission to any form of residential or institutional care implies that the individual has in some way broken out, or broken down, in his previous life (Berry, 1972). Older people coming into hospital or into residential care are coming from a situation of crisis or breakdown and experience a set of quantitative and qualitative losses. This is not to say that they have failed in their outside life: simply that they have come up against barriers that were insurmountable without help. Admission to care also implies a lack of suitable care in their own home.

Deprivation syndrome

There is now a considerable literature on the effects of loss, deprivation and distortion of relationships, especially of parenting relationships, on children. Bowlby (1951) produced the first influential attempt to bring together research on what has come to be known as 'maternal deprivation'. His original work rested heavily on the suggestion that the proper care of children deprived of a normal home life is not just an act of common humanity, but is essential for their mental and social welfare and that of the community. He deplored the treatment of children in institutions and the indifference to what he described as childish sensitivities and claimed that maternal deprivation could have grave and fundamental effects on a child's personality and intellect.

His views have been extremely influential, but his original claims about maternal deprivation have been much criticised, particularly on methodological grounds. Later research has begun to bring out the importance of physical and genetic factors in child development. Rutter (1972) identifies a number of points that can be taken for granted in the current state of knowledge. There is ample evidence that children show an immediate reaction of acute distress when admitted to hospital or to a residential nursery. Many infants do show retardation of development following admission to a low-grade institution and if left there for a long time they may show intellectual impairment. There is some association between delinquency and broken homes, and affectionless psychopathy sometimes follows multiple-separation experiences and institutional care in childhood.

Rutter goes on to suggest that the existence of the simple term 'maternal deprivation' tends to mask the fact that it includes a wide range of different experiences. Some of the evidence seems to point to the fact that adverse effects are not necessarily related to the mother and not necessarily to loss as such. The undesirable effects that institutions have on children may be related not to the loss of parental care that results but to the distortion of relationships and the lack of suitable substitute relationships that is often experienced. Later work by Bowlby (1969) emphasises the importance of attachment behaviour on the young child's need for continuing relationships with other people; this need is usually met through parents or parental figures. Rutter argues that distress probably arises partly through disruption of bonds, whereas affectionless psychopathy may tend to arise because firm bonds have never developed either through lack of available others or inadequacy of the relationships that were available.

This final point is of significance in a consideration of the applicability of findings on deprivation syndromes in children to long-term care of the elderly. Clearly the foundations of methods of coping with stress are learned in early life and the way older people respond to stress will be a reflection of the way mechanisms have been used in earlier life. Admission to care of the older person will cause a number of losses which might be expected to cause distress but it may also cause a distortion of relationships which might be expected to create particular problems.

Studies of older people and the effects of admission to institutions fall into two broad categories: those which examine the physical stress which occurs during and soon after admission and those which examine the nature of psychological and emotional effects.

In the former category a study by Kay, Norris and Post (1956) puts forward three factors that are prognostic of early death on admission to a psychiatric hospital: serious physical illness, acute organic confusional states, and age over 80. The presence of several of these signs increases the likelihood of early death. Rosin and Boyd (1966) found a high incidence of complications in elderly patients after admission to hospital. Complications unrelated to the illness precipitating the admission were as frequent as those associated with the original diagnosis; infections formed the largest group of incidental complications. A similar study by Reichel (1965) found a comparable rate of complications arising from hospital-caused factors and from intercurrent disease processes (also related to hospital factors: e.g. excessive bed-rest, inactivity, medication, dehydration).

Liebermann (1961) found that the relationship between physical status and mortality is more complex than this discussion might suggest. He suggests that the investigation of psychological aspects of death might be a fruitful area for research: if it can be shown that stress is a factor in early mortality then it may be possible to identify the more vulnerable patients.

Other studies have concentrated on psychological reactions to admission stress. Kent (1963) identifies some of the reasons for stress. Stress may arise when the resident realises that the 'parent surrogate' (hospital staff) has no intention of magically meeting all his needs. Disturbances before admission may be aggravated by a feeling of having been pressured by friends or relatives into applying for admission. The newly admitted resident may be unable to submit to a subordinate status.

Kent argues that response to stress may take a number of forms, from complete adjustment in a mature way on intellectual and emotional levels, through poor adjustment, to regression, rejection, paranoia and depression. Poor adjustment will involve feelings of being on the point of being engulfed, wandering, disorientation and restlessness, and even physical flight from the unbearable institutional situation.

Litin (1956) makes a much more explicit connection between the behaviour of children and older people on admission. He describes the child reacting in a terrified manner, certainly with apprehension and confusion. Overwhelming anxiety allows full rein to the child's fantasies and imaginings, especially at night. Many of these reactions are seen in older people admitted to hospital: delirium is common and, as with the child, this increases at night. Agitation, panic, aggression, destructiveness and incontinence are frequently seen and parallels can be drawn with the child's behaviour in similar circumstances.

A number of American studies have looked at the suggestion that relocation to special, age-segregated housing is undesirable because elderly people need contact with and stimulation from the young. Lawton (1970) found that while the amount of face-to-face contact with relatives tended to be reduced following a move from community housing to planned housing for the elderly there was no evidence that this was accompanied by a subjective feeling of estrangement from the family. Sherman (1975) found that residents of age-segregated housing tended to have less contact with children and families than older residents of dispersed housing but they had more new contacts and interacted more often with neighbours. She concluded that age-segregated housing does imply different spheres of contact and interaction but that either special housing or dispersed community housing can be satisfactory for the older person who feels he has freely made the choice to be there.

This element of 'felt rejection' is obviously of great importance in the relocation of older people. Ideally they should be able to look forward to positive elements of their new home. In reality they will often be experiencing stress either because of environmental inadequacies—poor housing, poverty, etc.—or because of relationship difficulties or poor health. It is particularly important, therefore, that all workers involved at this time develop skills in helping the older person through the move.

Admission to an institution can be seen to offer special hazards to people of all ages: loss of relationships and distortion of the bonds between people can lead to distress and emotional disturbance. In the case of older people these reactions are aggravated by increased vulnerability related to pre-admission crisis and in the case of hospital care by the dangers that lie within the hospital—infection, bad management of illness, limited activities, etc. The implications of this discussion for the provision of care are mainly in terms of the provision of adequate preparation before admission, careful handling of the admission process, preparation of the home or hospital beforehand, and the maintenance of familiar links in the new situation.

Some case examples illustrate the real problems of admissions to care which are insufficiently planned:

Mr C was 80 when he suffered a cerebral vascular accident which left him with a right hemiplegia. His wife was several years younger (67) and they had lived a quiet, happy life until that time. They had a son and daughter-in-law with three young children living nearby but no other relatives and few friends.

After one month's in-patient treatment Mr C returned home but attended a day hospital three times a week. Although his physical condition improved a little he was unable to co-operate very much in dressing himself or managing the toilet alone. Mrs C soon began to feel the physical strain of caring for him and this aggravated the strain in their interpersonal relationships. A social worker became involved and was able to give a lot of support to Mrs C who was relieved at the care and interest shown in her. In relieving Mrs C the social worker took some of the emotional pressure from Mr C who began to improve both physically and emotionally.

An arrangement was made for Mr C to be admitted for two weeks' in-patient care in the hospital he was familiar with while his wife went on holiday with their son. This unfortunately coincided with the social worker leaving the area. She took great care in introducing another social worker before she left and prepared Mr C for admission. The arrangements broke down when he was admitted to another, similar hospital without prior warning, for primarily administrative reasons.

He was bewildered by the sudden change and felt abandoned by his wife. When she returned from holiday he was apathetic, withdrawn, and had deteriorated so quickly that he was unfit to return home. The new social worker reported: 'eventually he seemed to recognize me but stared blankly at the wall throughout the interview. He showed no interest in me, in his wife, or in his return home: even mentioning the mix-up over the hospitals doesn't cause any spark' (on admission he had been very angry and suspicious).

Mr C never recovered from his withdrawal and he died a few weeks later, leaving his wife with a heavy burden of guilt.

Mr D's experience was less extreme than that of Mr C but followed a similar pattern. Always recognised as something of a local eccentric, by the time he had reached the age of 70 Mr D was living in a minute caravan in a friend's overgrown garden. He appeared to live on fish and chips and sweets and freely distributed the latter to local children. The caravan became very dilapidated and dirty, as did Mr D, whose health also began to deteriorate. However, he persisted in remaining in his caravan and was unfailingly cheerful. He had a ready, if rather repetitive, supply of jokes and songs performed for a spasmodic stream of visitors—mainly doctors, nurses, social workers and health visitors, all bent on persuading him to enter residential care.

He was eventually taken to a hospital assessment ward as an emergency after receiving burns when he set the caravan alight. On the ward he was subdued but quite cheerful until he learned he couldn't go back to the caravan which had been badly damaged. He was eventually admitted to a residential home where the staff described him as 'a nice old man, but I can't see what all the fuss was about'. The social worker, visiting him a fortnight after admission reported: 'he was sitting by himself in his bedroom looking clean and well fed. He didn't mention the first world war at all.' Bewildered by events which had moved outside his control Mr D felt flattened and overwhelmed. He withdrew into a passive shell and was never able to reassert his individuality.

55

Preparing the client—the geriatric team

One important way of overcoming some of the difficulties that have been described is by making adequate, careful preparation before admission. This will involve the worker in the community in making a full assessment of client needs in order to be sure that admission is the best course of action and in discussion and clarification of the implications of admission to build up strengths before the event. If the problems of the elderly are multi-symptomatic then the 'solutions' to those problems will best be found by a team of workers both in the community and in the hospital or residential environment. Social workers, health visitors, nurses, general practitioners and hospital doctors all become involved with the older person and his family and friends. Considerable change is often brought about in client's lives by team intervention and it is important to be aware of the implications of the intervention of the geriatric team for social change.

Geriatric medicine is concerned perhaps as much with the continuing management of illness and future health care of elderly patients as with the treatment of presenting illness. This concern inevitably extends to the social and emotional needs of the individual patient who can only remain independent in terms of his total internal and external environment. In some senses bringing about change in the life of an elderly patient, a client and his family, with limited material resources, is a daunting prospect, particularly in the face of a limited capacity for personal change within the individual. From a different standpoint the changes that can take place are very fundamental. An elderly person can be removed from complete independence to total dependence by a crisis illness or can be moved from a safe, warm, caring hospital environment to a lonely, isolated existence in a cold, damp house.

It is important, therefore, to bear in mind that perceptions of the nature and extent of the change that takes place are often very different. What looks like an ideal solution to the doctor, social worker or the anxious relative, may look like a fate worse than death to the older person. Bringing about social change is not necessarily a desirable objective but is usually an inevitable result of intervention by members of the geriatric team. It is important also to look carefully at who is bringing about the change, why it is being brought about and in which area of the client's functioning the change is taking place. The usual tasks of the social worker have been seen as bringing about change in the older person's material environment by direct social intervention and helping the elderly individual make attitudinal adjustments to changed physical, environmental and interpersonal circumstances. This concept of the social-work role must be very carefully examined in relation to the overall operation of the geriatric team. In addition to his own personal and professional attitudes and values each member of the team brings to the change situation a range of helping techniques that rests on a particular set of theoretical constructs. These helping skills will be applied in terms of the implicit and explicit tasks and objectives of the agency within which the work is being carried out. It is plain that the geriatric team members hold many of these factors in common: it is equally plain that in many cases it will be the doctor, nurse or health visitor who will bring about personal or social change.

The social worker cannot hold a monopoly as the agent of social change. An elderly person can be seen as functioning within a number of social systems. The introduction of a new person into any of these social systems inevitably leads to adjustments in the pattern of the client's or patient's life. Each member of the team contributes new facets to the patient's life and part of the social worker's role is the interpretation of the patient's social functioning to the rest of the team and the organisation and direction of their individual interventions towards agreed social objectives.

It is important for the team to reach an assessment of social data and to establish a set of objectives for the personal and social development of the elderly person in need. A medical approach to a problem will have as its final objectives the restoration of an optimum level of functioning. The solutions to 'social problems' have very often not taken into account the continuing needs of the older person. To put an old lady into an old people's home may meet the immediate need for physical care, but without additional provisions for emotional support, continuing family contact, and regular reviews of her needs, it will not be a solution.

Social interventions must take account of the fact that ageing is a process (or a collection of processes) and must aim to provide ongoing care that will leave room for the developing needs of each individual. The social-work contribution to the team's understanding of this developing need will be an interpretation of the patient's or client's previous social and emotional development (how he has become the kind of person he is), of the way he views his current predicaments, and of the way his attitudes to his illness, his family, the ageing process, etc., will influence his future functioning in society.

The social worker in the community

In so far as they provide new and different relationships for the older person and in so far as they function within the same community or hospital system all members of the geriatric team contribute to changing the patient's or client's life. It is therefore vitally important that each member of the geriatric team is made aware, and remains aware, of the impact of his own interaction on the older person's social functioning. Nevertheless the community social worker is the one professional whose primary aim is relief of stress in social situations through a flexible use of personal and community resources.

Social work is rapidly developing and it needs much clarification. The social worker will be involved in direct and indirect intervention with the patient, his family, the social systems within which he lives and the internal institutional organisation as well as the wide, formal and informal organisations in the community. The form which the intervention is likely to take will vary widely. An early reliance on a casework approach, which drew heavily on psycho-dynamic theories, has been supplemented by a growing interest in community-work and group-work approaches. This growth of interest is closely linked to a growth in the demand for a range of social action that will recognise the pressures on individual need of the wide environmental spectrum of poverty and deprivation. Social work discussion has reflected this growing demand for new ideas. At one end of the spectrum casework has been precisely defined as (Younghusband, 1959, p. 55):

> a continuous professional relationship, a process of dynamic interaction between worker and client consciously used for social treatment purposes defined by a study of the particular person in his situation, the problems which most concern him and the ways he could be helped to meet these by the use of his own and the community's resources.

Other writers have emphasised the fact that poverty and deprivation are a structural problem of society (Burton, 1974, p. 462):

> Social economic, and political structures that create and main-tain inequalities of income and opportunity reflected in educa-tional systems and employment, are a fundamental cause of poverty and deprivation . . . it is social workers that shoulder the main responsibility of seeing something is done about poverty and deprivation.

The social worker's intervention will take many forms, from the provision of home helps or residential care to the use of casework skills or stimulating social action. In a time of such rapid develop-ment in social work it is hardly surprising that consumers and colleagues in other caring professions find it hard to identify the task of the social worker.

Some central elements in the task of the field social worker in relation to the admission of an old person to residential care can be identified. Each client has a right to a full and careful assessment of his individual needs. In order to carry out this assessment the social worker must collect basic data which will be relevant in terms of the decisions that must be made. There are two decisions to be made in assessment: what is the problem with which the client needs help, and what is the action that could be taken. In relation to admission to residential care this means reaching a decision with the client on the nature of the blocks to the progress of a satisfactory life and on the appropriateness of residential care as a way of surmounting the blocks.

There may sometimes be a tendency to perceive and present problems in terms of available, identifiable resources. It is easier to say 'I need an old people's home' than to say 'I need help but I don't know what kind of help'. The first point in assessment in this case is to disentangle the problem from the resources and redefine it in more realistic terms. Clear assessment is further complicated by a process of 'crisis inertia' (Brearley, 1972) whereby neighbours perceive the older person in difficulties and pass on an exaggerated perception of the difficulties to the health visitor, general practitioner, etc., who add their own perceptions. The 'crisis' that is finally presented to the social worker as an emergency may bear little resemblance to the real needs of the elderly client.

In order to gather information the social worker needs to be able to communicate with the old person—who may present special problems of deafness, poor sight, dementia, etc.—and with others in the community. Communication may be verbal or non-verbal; it may be through words or tone of voice, or through facial expression or actions. To recognise the meaning of a message may take time and patience (particularly true of the geriatric patient) and it is essential to create an environment of trust in which the client feels free to express himself.

At the centre of the social worker's task is the controlled understanding and use of relationships. The relationship may occasionally be used to promote new understandings of attitudes and behaviour but will mainly be aimed at providing opportunities to reflect on current environmental pressures, to look for satis-factions in the total pattern of the client's life, and to present material resources in a flexible and sensitive way. In examining the effectiveness of social work with elderly clients Goldberg (1970) emphasised the importance of environmental and practical support of all kinds, particularly for those living alone or with limited family resources. The importance of reaching out and holding on to clients was highlighted, as was the enabling and supporting role of the social worker with the elderly. This study also found that reassuring and emotionally satisfying reminiscences can help the old person regain a sense of positive worth and identity. Above all the study strikingly demonstrated the importance and validity of a careful and sound initial assessment.

The social worker in preparing the older person for admission to care has several important tasks. He must make a thorough assessment and both he and the client should be sure it is the most appropriate course of action. He must give the client time to communicate his real feelings and make sure that the client understands the reality of the proposed move. Understanding this reality will certainly involve visiting the new home, perhaps staying there for a little while whenever possible. Too often older people are given inadequate information and explanation, driven through unfamiliar countryside to a home that wasn't built the last time they were able to get out of the house. Having clarified the reality of the move the worker must facilitate discussion of feelings about the move: a certain amount of discussion of anxieties before admission may facilitate adjustment later.

Perhaps most important of all is the social worker's role in helping the client with material, practical difficulties of housing, tenancies, disposal or storage of furniture, etc. One consideration to be borne in mind at this time is whether it is realistic to keep open a way out from residential care. The caring system of hospital/old people's home/sheltered housing can be described as a funnel which is too small to take in the number of old people who need help. There are at least three ways of relieving congestion at the mouth of the funnel: by increasing the number of beds available, by increasing the provision of domiciliary services, and by widening the exit to the funnel. If more people move through and out of the system more can be accommodated. It is therefore always necessary to consider leaving open ways out where practical and to build in regular reviews of the needs of older people in care. To the community social worker residential care should be a resource to be used carefully and flexibly and only after a full assessment in conjunction with the residential worker. Residential care is just one therapeutic resource in a wide range of possibilities and certainly need not be either the first resort or a last resort.

There are, of course, problems for the social worker in using residential resources, which are aggravated by limited domiciliary resources and increasing community pressures. The discussion of the objectives of institutional care has already pointed to the complexity of aims: institutions have the widely different aims of treatment, containment, protection, etc., which are all likely to exist to a greater or lesser extent in each institution. The conflict and confusion of aims may also exist in the social worker and cause anxieties and uncertainties about actions. Sometimes the anxiety is dealt with by pushing away responsibility, and procedures become very formalised and inflexible (form-filling, etc.) and responsibility is pushed upwards in a departmental hierarchy. There is also a strong authority content in some uses of residential care, which may lead to anxiety and uncertainty. In addition difficulties result from handling over the client, even partly, to another worker on admission to care: the 'Whose child is this?' conflict is equally relevant to the care of the elderly.

The social worker's role lies in smoothing the practicalities of admission and in helping the client towards a realistic handling of fantasies.

Preparing the home—the residential worker's role

The last mentioned difficulty of the field worker in handing over a client exists as a difficulty also for the residential worker. It is often hard to share clients but it is important for the smooth arrangement of admission that field and residential workers can collaborate. Just as it is important for the client to visit the home it may in some situations be important for the residential worker to visit the old person in his own home before admission. Whether this is useful for a particular client must be a matter for discussion between field worker, client and residential worker: some clients feel happier if they can meet the new worker on safe ground where they feel able to present their whole personality. The field worker's assessment must be available to the residential worker who must know how to follow up the existing treatment programme, or how to modify it and, in the short term, how to prepare the home for the client.

Preparations will be on the practical level and on individual and group levels in the home. The new resident should feel he is expected and welcomed: the fears and fantasies about the home will only be exaggerated by inadequate preparation for arrival:

Mrs E was to be admitted to a home for two weeks while her family went on holiday. The social worker took her to visit the home and helped her to think about the difficulties beforehand so that if she was not looking forward to the stay she at least accepted the idea calmly. On the morning of the admission the social worker took Mrs E to the home as arranged and found that an old man had been admitted to the bed as an emergency the previous night. Mrs E had to go to another home, quite near, but totally strange to her: the social worker reported: 'She was much more nervous and she was pale and quiet in the car on the way.'

61

Entering care

> When they arrived at the second home the room was not ready and Mrs E had to sit on a hard chair in the corridor waiting for the bed to be made.

Not only was she distressed and disorientated by the sudden, unavoidable change of plans but the nature of her reception left much to be desired, as the social worker described:

> 'When the bed was made the attendant picked up her case and said, "Is this all, dear?" She then unpacked the case, calling out each item as she put them away in a drawer. All the time this was going on Mrs E sat out in the corridor, on the verge of tears.'

After their arrival most old people need a period of quiet to settle themselves in with some privacy. There must, however, be a balance between privacy and isolation and the resident group has a right to know who is joining them and the newcomer has a right to be introduced. The initial impression is very important:

> Miss F was admitted to hospital suffering from hypothermia. She had no family and the house was in a very poor state. When she recovered she applied for admission to residential care and was eventually offered accommodation. The young, male social worker took her home to collect some clothes since she had only night clothes and dressing gown. She was able to collect a few things but these were in a poor state after being in the empty house for several months. The social worker could give her little help and she reached the home looking very untidy and down-at-heel. She was highly conscious of this and although the staff quickly solved the problem she never felt that she could overcome the initial impression she created. In fact two other residents were actually heard to say, some weeks later, 'She's all right now but you should have seen the state she was in when she arrived.'

Entering any new group causes anxiety: entering a closed group with the very strict boundaries of the institution creates considerable anxiety. Each new resident brings his own individual needs to take things from and to give back to the group. The initial task of the residential worker is to reduce the practical difficulties to a minimum and to help the old person into the institutional group.

Hospital care—the sick role

Entering residential care requires special adjustment but entry to hospital has the added requirement of making an adaptation to being ill. The role of sick person may be recently acquired or it may

62

be longstanding and it carries with it certain expectations which will be emphasised by admission to hospital.

The concept of role has diverse origins. Parsons (1951) said that role is 'that organized sector of an actor's orientation which constitutes and defines his participation in an interactive process. It involves a set of complementary expectations concerning his own actions and those of others with whom he interacts.' Many definitions stress the unitary nature of roles: Levinson (1959) suggests three points that are emphasised in definitions. Role may be defined as the structurally given demands (norms, taboos, responsibilities) associated with a given social position; it may be defined as the conception of the individual of the part he is going to play in the organisation; and role may also be defined as the actions of the individual organisation members. The unitary conception of role assumes a high degree of congruence between these three but this is not necessarily so (Morris, 1971).

Bates (1956) develops four useful postulates concerning role and status (or position). First, he argues that within any given culture there is a limited number of roles which combine in various ways to compose a limited number of positions. Second, within any given position there tends to be a strain towards consistency or adjustment between the various roles composing a position. Third, each position contains certain dominant roles to which are adjusted certain recessive roles. Finally, no role exists without a paired reciprocal role which is part of a different position.

Parsons proposes a conceptual framework which may provide a basis to review the behaviour of the elderly sick. He makes a number of assumptions: role is an individual's performance of differentiated tasks within his social system; illness, or disability, produces incapacity and limits or inhibits the performance of tasks. Health, on the other hand, represents a state of optimum capacity for the performance of valued tasks. Similarly rehabilitation refers to any treatment or service which is aimed at restoring or optimising capacity for the appropriate performance of role-tasks. Illness or disability also disrupts the role-patterns of the family and permanent illness leads to a reorganisation of the family social system. In relation to American values Parsons makes four behavioural assumptions about the sick role: the sick person is exempt from social responsibility; the sick person cannot be expected to take care of himself; the sick person should want to get well; the sick person should seek medical advice and co-operate with medical experts. Although some of these points can be criticised as not strictly relevant to chronic sickness or disability they do provide a foundation for discussion.

Illness or disability may cause extreme anxiety: the sick role may be rejected and individual reactions may follow a variety of pathological patterns (denial, regression, withdrawal, etc.). Levinson (1959) suggests that adaptation to role-conflict may be in any one of a number of ways. The individual may change his role-conception and adapt his personality to the organisation: the way the elderly patient learns to play the sick role in the hospital is partly a function of his relationships with caring staff and other patients. The individual may alternatively leave the organisation; this is not often a solution for the elderly patient. Alternatively he may remain, but in a state of apathetic conformity, meeting the minimal requirements of role-performance: this is a familiar picture of the long-stay elderly patient. A further mode of adaptation is to gain sufficient power to change the organisation; the importance of participation of patients in their own care will be discussed fully later.

On an individual psychological level Storr (1960b) describes two broad forms of adaptation to the sick role. He suggests that the attitudes of adults to illness are derivatives of their attitudes towards adults in childhood. The more introvert person treats illness as an attack from without, fears the restrictions imposed by illness: in its extreme form this reaction is paranoid and obsessive. This kind of patient is inclined to ask the question 'Why should this happen to me?' but he is likely to put up a better fight against the illness. The extroverted patient feels that his helpless condition calls for support: he is likely to become dependent and to tend towards a depressive reaction. The question he asks is 'What have I done wrong to deserve this?' and his attitude is generally a passive, dependent one.

Following this kind of analysis it is interesting to speculate whether long-stay patients in geriatric hospitals are more likely to belong to the latter grouping: those who fight illness and caring staff may be more likely to get out into the community again. It may, correspondingly, be that elderly patients in a dependent, passive position have a reserve capacity for improvement which might be described as reflecting chronic adaptation.

The sick role and chronic adaptation in the elderly

Blau (1973) argues that serious consideration should be given to the proposition that 'illness' has a psychological function for older people in modern societies. Since society has no clearly defined role for the elderly, sickness may serve as a socially acceptable way of legitimising this rolelessness. The sick role may provide the old person with special rights and privileges and act as a defence against the ego threat of rolelessness. There is evidence (Birren, 1972) that the older nervous system has a reserve plasticity which, by inference, may show a characteristic level of activity that may reflect in part chronic adaptation. This impairment of adaptation may result from relative sensory deprivation resulting from diminishing environmental stimulation which is often a concomitant of ageing and which will be aggravated by increasing loss of hearing and sight. The level of physical activity in old age seems to be very important to positive adaptation. Gore (1972) has reviewed Russian literature on this subject and describes work which demonstrates that physical exercise in elderly subjects can improve health.

Chronic adaptation can be seen as the result of two related factors. To some extent it is the result of an under-use of existing faculties which may result from psychological and environmental factors and it may also arise out of a failure to utilise alternative abilities to compensate for illness-related losses. Chronic adaptation is a concept that can relate to physical, emotional and social adjustments and is usually the result of unsuitable environment. In order to draw on the reserve capacity that chronic adaptation implies, it will be necessary to provide stimuli directed at the development of new coping mechanisms and the extension of existing methods. At every level of the individual organisation adaptive mechanisms develop as a result of internal and external change. Froimovich and Acle (1972) suggest that people do not become unadapted simply because they have lived a certain number of years: they propose the use of the term 'social relocation' instead of social adaptation. Most people, they argue, retain a high percentage of capacities which can be relocated to permit them to live a useful life in society.

This relocation of capacities will follow, in the hospital and residential-settings, from an increase in stimulation and motivation. The ways in which social institutions provide a supportive 'social climate' and are orientated towards social responsibilities in dealing with life crises of older people are critical in understanding the phenomena of social adaptation (Beattie, 1972). An understanding of sick-role behaviour and the special needs of older people which often lead to a degree of chronic adaptation is essential for the provision of appropriate support, stimulation, and motivation in hospital and residential care.

Entering care—a summary

Older people going into hospital or an old people's home will experience loss and deprivation, which will cause stress and distortion of relationships, which may cause maladaptation. Responses to stress are aggravated by increased risk of infection and hospital-related illness. Difficulties are likely to be related to the availability, or non-availability, of good substitute relationships in the community group. Workers in the geriatric team of the hospital, the residential home and the community can reduce the extent of the stress by working together to prepare the client or patient emotionally and practically. It is essential also that the institution is adequately prepared and above all that support is given at the point of admission.

In a report produced in 1975 for the Personal Social Services Council on living and working in residential homes it was argued that a clearly worded contract should be agreed between the resident of a home and the providing authority. A prospectus would give the resident outline information of the service to be provided and the resident would agree to the various rules of the home and other conditions. The important implication is that the elements of care would be spelled out explicitly at the beginning of care. In addition to this the report also highlights the importance of a carefully planned programme of continuing care with stated objectives agreed between residents, their family and the staff.

The point of admission is a vitally important time for setting the standard for care: much more time and effort needs to be devoted to the development of skills and approaches if residential care is to be used to its full potential in the future. A recognition of the existence of a reserve capacity for growth in the older person is essential to the development of skills in the use of appropriate stimulation, support, motivation, etc.

Chapter five

Working with the individual in the communal group

The fundamental problem of any individual, at any age, admitted to any institution, is the conflict between the need to feel safe, secure and wanted and the need to remain an independent, integrated, whole person. In the old people's home the residential worker is concerned with maintaining a balance between these two needs. The principal aim in doing this will be to provide, on an individual level, a secure environment in which the older person can recover from the crisis of admission and the problems that preceded it, to initiate and sustain a process of holding and support which maintains a satisfying, continuing life, and in which growth and development are at the least a possibility.

Integration and repair

Most if not all the old people who come into care do so as a result of some crisis in their home. This may have been an environmental problem (poor housing, increasing brain failure leading to deteriorating standards, etc.), a relationship problem (insufficient supports, family stress, etc.) or a problem of physical illness or increasing disability. The elderly individual is therefore coming into a strange environment at a time of low personal strengths. It may well be that he has been battered into a state of apathetic withdrawal from the world and his first need is for the repair of the damage that has been done.

One primary need in residential situations is for good physical care, which will include warmth, food and comfortable surroundings. It is important to bear in mind, in this connection, that perceptions of comfort may vary. An old person coming from a home made up of old but familiar furniture may see a brand new, purpose-built and designed environment as bare and unwelcoming;

most older people have been used to coal fires and may also find centrally heated homes less satisfying. It is important also not to become too involved in stressing the physical comforts of the home. A home or ward full of clean, well-fed, neatly clothed bodies can be a much less comfortable and comforting environment than one which is less spotless or less neat and tidy but which has recognisably individual people living in it. Physical care, however, is an essential prerequisite to the process of recovery after admission. If strength has been over-expended on the struggle to survive in the community it must be rebuilt before full adjustment to communal living can begin. When staff are involved in providing the basic necessities of life they are also involved in providing one of the fundamental elements in the parental role. The parent is the provider and children are dependent on this provision for their growth. It is likely that in the first stages of life in the home some older people will regress in their behaviour and accept some elements of the child's role.

Dependence can be a growth experience for the older person. Many older people, especially those who need residential care, have outlived those who provided them with love and affection. The need to be wanted is an important part of finding contentment in life and the residential worker, who is in such close contact with the resident throughout the day and night, may have to meet this need, at least in an initial phase. This process might be described as 'holding'. Normally, holding the elderly resident will mean demonstrating in practical ways as well as verbally that he is valued and valuable and on occasions it will involve physical touch. Reaching out is an essential part of holding.

Staff will need to demonstrate their feeling that all residents are valued for their individual worth, and that they are accepted as whole people. This involves an acceptance of the whole person, including his unpleasant, unsociable, regressive habits. Some residents may indulge in these as a way of testing the staff's real attitudes. Regression may take the form of incontinence, bad table manners, or even temporary confusion and wandering. If residents are allowed a period of regression, and indulgence in simply being cared for, then they will have the chance to build up physical and emotional strengths and be able to release energies for self-maintenance and growth activities.

This is not, of course, to suggest that all residents need to regress, nor is it a suggestion that self-indulgence is necessarily desirable; it is merely a proposition that a recovery period is essential after admission. Although this recovery period is a time to allow residents to build up strengths, it is also a time to set limits on them. One important part of running a residential home is the balanced use of authority to promote group and individual satisfactions. The resident group will impose some checks and balances on the behaviour of individuals but sometimes staff will have to use additional controls. In the initial period following admission these controls are an important part of regulating and balancing the extent of dependence and regression: external controls keep the individual in touch with reality. A positive sense of authority will arise from contact with a worker who treats the residents with a consistent respect and who explores with individual residents their feelings about the limitations that are being put on them.

A further important element in the recovery and integration process for new residents is the need for protection. In one sense this means providing safety regulations, or rules that will provide for the physical well-being of staff and residents. This will include rules about smoking in bed, about use of stairs, lifts, etc., but it is imperative that these rules are flexible and are clearly discussed and agreed with each individual. Rules should not infringe personal liberty and personal controls should come from within the individual resident. Workers must sometimes be prepared to take risks. A short life but a merry one may be a good alternative to a long but miserable life. In a second sense it may be necessary to provide some protection for the new resident from the rest of the resident group. For most people this will involve practical issues of helping them learn about group expectations—where to sit, how to behave, etc.—and helping them in the exploration of possible roles in the group. The key factor in protection of residents should be flexibility of approach: treating all residents in the same way may not be fair treatment. An individual approach to individual need is vital.

The residential worker should aim, then, to provide the new resident with a secure foundation from which to view the world at a safe distance. After a period of crisis the resident needs to build up his strengths and to do this he may need to become inward-looking and regressive. Only after he has concentrated on himself will he be able to look outwards for a new life in the communal group.

Holding and maintenance

If the resident's first need is for a period of building up strengths his continuing need is to be able to maintain a contented life, which will involve making an adaptation to his new surroundings. The provision of security and physical care and comfort must continue as a prerequisite of adaptation. Although 'holding' the elderly resident may be a recurring need it is important for the residential worker to be aware of the difficulties and dangers of over-dependence. Individuals can, and do, build up strengths and can experience personal growth through a dependent relationship but there are limitations on dependence as a growth experience. In this context some comments on psychoanalytical considerations will be useful.

Object-relations theory (Klein, 1960) proposes that in very early infancy feelings are less mixed than in later life: loving and hating are kept separate. Through the relationship with the mother, or the mother's breast—the most significant part of her to the infant—the child learns to invest the object with the feeling he is experiencing. In this way the mother is a 'good object' when she gives food and other satisfactions and a 'bad object' when she removes or withholds the satisfactions. The good and bad objects and feelings therefore exist in the child's inner and outer reality and as the child grows and perceives that his mother is a separate individual, good and bad feelings are integrated and introjected in his inner world and the two opposing feelings can be held about the same object. Ambivalence is one element in all relationships and situations and at times of anxiety and stress there may be a tendency to split good and bad feelings and project them on to others in the environment. Dependent relationships of elderly residents may encourage this kind of splitting and residential workers may find themselves being cast as evil, or in ideal terms.

The concept of transference implies the transfer of feelings more appropriate to earlier relationships on to someone in the current environment. In the case of the elderly resident or patient this would involve him holding feelings towards the residential worker that he originally felt towards his parents. It may also be that the residential worker is not treated as a parent but as a son, daughter, husband or wife: this can be seen, in fact, as a transference reaction once removed. In the transference situation the alternative attitudes of clinging to others for support and protection but reacting with anger and avoidance when independence is threatened are reproduced (Storr, 1960a). Although both attitudes are present it is usual for one to predominate. It is arguable that there are elements of transference in all relationships and it is easy to see that the dependence which may result from close contact in a residential situation is likely to encourage this kind of reaction. Transference implies an unreal perception of, and reaction to, the worker, and the residential worker must be constantly aware of the likelihood of its occurrence. He should also be aware of the possibility of his acceptance of the implied parental role—counter-transference. A comprehensive treatment of these concepts is given by Isca Salzberger-Wittenberg (1970).

If the residential worker is conscious of playing a parenting role and can use it to help the resident build up his personal strengths for a limited period then dependence and transference may be useful tools. They should not be over-used: over-dependence will lead to idealisation or angry avoidance of the worker—neither of which is helpful to the resident.

It has been suggested in an earlier chapter that satisfaction may be associated with the opportunity to achieve ego integrity. By the time people have reached old age they are firmly established as individuals: no major personality changes will take place. Some rebuilding and repair of the personality will follow from a controlled use of dependence but for most elderly residents the major task is concerned with ego adaption. Whether they view the present and future with resignation, with fear and anxiety, or with acceptance and satisfaction is likely to be related to their perception of a total pattern in their lives. One important task of the residential worker will be to ensure that each resident has the opportunity to review his situation. To do this he must be able to build a relationship which will contain elements of trust that will allow the resident to reflect on his current situation, on the totality of his past life, and on the immediate past—on the reasons for his being in the home or hospital. If the older person is able to see a meaningful and inevitable pattern in his life this may help him towards an acceptance of the present and the future. This is not an easy task: many older people in care have a memory impairment, others show a pattern of chronic brain failure, and others are unable, for very realistic reasons, to find meaning in their lives. Nevertheless, sharing of thoughts and ideas will help to clarify feelings and attitudes and reminiscence has the real value of enabling older people to look into their past lives for positive coping methods to use in the present. Self-expression through discussion is valuable and may sometimes be met by the worker and at other times through relationships between residents. The residential worker should encourage and stimulate the development of relationships within the resident group wherever possible.

The maintenance of a continuing pattern of life is therefore dependent on the capacity to regain personality strengths after admission and on the availability of caring relationships through which residents can achieve a reflective consideration of past, present and future, and achieve self-expression through mutual support and interaction. The maintenance of self-esteem and the self-concept is largely dependent on the existence of these opportunities for reflection and interaction.

Integrity and growth

The limitations of personality growth in the elderly have been pointed out. Many old people, however, might expect to live in an old people's home for several years, even for as long as ten or fifteen years. This is quite a considerable span of life and it would be wrong to assume that the pattern of life will remain static throughout the whole stay: some movement and change is inevitable, and desirable. Residents should be allowed the opportunity for decision-making: the importance of choice in providing care has already been described and the process of exercising choice in making decisions is a necessary part of self-direction and the achievement of personal integrity. Simple basic decisions about privacy during dressing, times for going to bed, etc. will give the resident a feeling of being in control of at least a part of his life and bring a related feeling of self-direction.

The residential worker should be able to use relationships with individual residents to promote increased activity and stimulate the achievement of new satisfactions. The element of positive control that continues to demonstrate a flexible respect for the individual, and the careful acceptance of a limited degree of dependence to provide support at times of particular stress, are important parts of the use of a relationship. The worker must also accept the elderly resident for his value as an individual while not necessarily approving of his behaviour in any particular situation: at times of stress the worker should try to understand how the resident feels, without becoming caught up in the resident's own distress or panic. In being continuously aware of his relationships with residents the worker can help to create an environment in which they can accept practical help, as well as allowing them to express strong feelings and accept the situation realistically. Occasionally it may be possible to facilitate the residents achieving insight into their own needs and behaviour. Additionally, in the group situation the worker can help to identify the processes and interaction of the group and can use the group to help individuals within it. Residents will often use relationships with other residents to provide this service: a few are unable to build relationships themselves, or are unable to use friends to help overcome particular problems and will need extra support.

One other way in which the elderly resident can be helped to extend his functioning is in the development of community and family links. Relatives of elderly residents or patients often feel guilty at not caring for them at home and this guilt is expressed both in over-visiting and in under-visiting, as well as in over-anxiety about, for example, the feeding and diet of the old person, and sometimes in hostility towards residential staff. It is as much a part of the residential worker's task to help the relatives to cope realistically with these feelings as it is to protect the resident from their effects. If the institution can be extended into the community and the community, especially relatives of residents, can be encouraged to come into the institution, then the range of available roles and relationships, and their attendant advantages, will also be extended.

On an individual level, then, the residential worker is concerned with helping the elderly resident with repair of damage caused before, and by, admission, with the maintenance of a satisfying pattern of daily life, and with providing stimulation, support and opportunities for extension of interest and functioning as individual needs change and develop. In achieving these objectives there are some special needs that will have to be considered.

Special needs

The need for privacy is a very important aspect of care, although it should be remembered that the words 'privacy' and 'privation' share a common root. In a practical sense privacy will involve leaving the individual resident enough freedom from interference for him to exercise personal choice in decision-making. Some residents may wish to share a room but most will prefer to be alone and to put an individual stamp on their own room with personal items, photographs, etc. Other residents may, in fact, prefer to share with three or four other people rather than be alone, or in a situation of enforced intimacy with only one other person. Privacy must be an essentially personal concept: for some people being alone is desirable, for others it may lead to loneliness. Loneliness in an institutional group is related not to the availability of contacts so much as to the elderly person's capacity to use the relationships that are available. The residential worker can help to overcome this and should always be conscious of the distinction between the wish for privacy when bathing, dressing, resting, etc., and withdrawal into hiding from interaction.

Residential workers should also be aware of the sexual needs of elderly residents. The popular view of sexual activity is closely tied up with ideas about romantic love and about physical beauty and attractiveness. The stereotyped attitude towards continued sexual activity in the elderly (perhaps also linked with children's attitudes to parental sexual activities) is that it is at best unusual and at worst unhealthy and even deviant. Studies (Kinsey, Pomeroy and Martin, 1948; Masters and Johnson, 1966; Pfeiffer, Verwoerdt and Wang, 1968) have shown that a substantial number of men and women continue to engage in sexual activity well beyond the age of 60. Although it is generally accepted that frequency of sexual intercourse declines with increasing age, the continuance of sexual activity is closely linked to the availability of a partner and the maintenance of an unbroken relationship.

Working with the individual in the communal group

Many factors influence sexual behaviour in the older person: attitudes of family, friends, neighbours, church and community are all likely to play a part. The woman may feel more relaxed after the menopause when she need no longer fear pregnancy but the older man tends to place sexual intercourse low on his list of priorities after retirement (Finkle, 1971). Increased contact after retirement may dull sexual interest as may drugs, alcohol and inactivity during the day. The attitudes of children and family, and also the general practitioner, are also influential. If the doctor reacts with surprise this may confirm suspicions that intercourse is dangerous to health. The attitudes of residential workers will have a similar effect.

A few married couples are admitted to residential care, and others marry during residence: their need for a private sex life should be respected and accepted. Most residents are either widowed or single but they may still wish for the company of the opposite sex, in a general way, and this should be encouraged and treated as normal, not ridiculed. The sexual need is a basic drive and if it is not satisfied tensions result. Some people are able to sublimate their energies into creative directions, others may need help in directing their energies constructively.

It is important also to be aware of the individual's need for a right to personal property and to retain control over his own finances. The hospital patient is particularly likely to be in a deprived position from this point of view. Often unable to spend money he may accumulate savings but because of organisational mechanisms be unable to gain access to them. Patients and residents should be free to decide how, when and where their money is to be spent or otherwise disposed of. This must be much more than a token gesture of obtaining a signature with a brief explanation. They should have free access and should be able easily to withdraw or deposit money.

Often patients in hospital have few clothes of their own and sometimes this is true in old people's homes. Inadequate laundry facilities and low staffing levels contribute to this and it seems essential to maintaining self-respect that older people in institutions should be able to decide which of their own clothes to wear. Similarly there should be separate places in which personal possessions can be kept—a private area which the individual can identify as his own with furniture, photographs, etc. In reality this may not be possible, or only in a limited way because of the need for protection: mental frailty sometimes precludes some residents from controlling their money and may also lead to intrusion on to others in the form of wandering, pilfering, etc. Nevertheless the need for individual protection should not be used as an excuse for deprivation of the freedom to make decisions about personal property.

74

Working with the individual in the communal group

The great majority of old people who live in an institutional setting will also die there. Death and dying are a common part of life in care and different establishments find different ways of handling this. Family and individual dignity should be respected in the way death and burial arrangements are handled. In residential care the stress is perhaps more to be placed on death than on the process of dying: residents either experience a brief terminal phase or they are admitted to hospital for longer-term care. Most elderly residents will feel a need to talk about death at some time and to review their feelings about the approach of death. Some will say that they are ready for death, that they feel that they have lived a good and useful life and they are 'ready to go'. 'I wish he'd come and take me' is a not uncommon comment and sometimes this kind of reaction may seem quite realistic. It may, however, be that this is a depressive form of reaction and that what seems like a calm acceptance of the reality, may be apathetic depression. With treatment for the depression interest in life may be renewed. Once again the residential worker must learn to distinguish realistic acceptance, which can be encouraged by individual and group discussion (when the residents make this possible), from depression.

In hospital, and to a rather less common extent in residential care, the dying patient should continue to be treated as a whole person and not just as a dying body. If the doctor on his ward-round passes by the bed, or if the patient is moved into a single ward, this will emphasise feelings of rejection. Anxiety and mental distress in the dying patient tend to be associated with physical distress (Hinton, 1963) and successful treatment of the physical aspects of distress will always ease the emotional reaction (Saunders, 1967). The threat of pain leads to tension and anxiety in the patient and his family and if this threat can be removed they can be helped to relax and to cope with the emotional reaction. Saunders stresses the value of listening and communication, creative activity and ordinary social interchange in helping to ease the loneliness of the dying person. Helping the dying will require an ability to be aware of the patient's feelings about death and to separate these from the worker's own fears. It is no help to say, 'I know how you feel. If I were you I would be terrified.' It may be helpful to say, 'I think I know how you feel but I care enough to help you with your fears.'

Death in most hospitals, and some residential homes, is coped with in ritualised, standardised ways. Sometimes a more significant member of the communal group dies and leaves a major gap and the group must go through a period of grieving for their joint loss. The worker should be able to help them in their grieving and encourage them to see the loss in a realistic context.

The individual in the group

The individual who arrives in the institutional group will bring with him all the needs that have been described. Above all he will need to be recognised as a person and he will need to influence and affect others within the group. He will have a picture of how he would like to be seen by others and will seek to impose that image on the group that he is joining. In fact he is not joining just one group but a number of people who will form different groups for different purposes. The resident group as a whole is unlikely to meet together very often, except for the purpose of meals. At other times residents are likely to split themselves into groups who use different sitting rooms, or who come together to watch television or to attend a handicraft session, etc. Each of these groups will have a different pattern of interaction and will have a separate set of norms and conventions. The new resident will have to learn to adapt to each of these groups, which may change in their composition and patterns of interaction simply because of his arrival within the group.

He will be expected to conform to simple sets of rules and expectations. All residential workers are familiar with the fact that most elderly residents have a special chair and if the newcomer inadvertently sits in the wrong place this can cause an argument which may rankle for long afterwards. These expectations can be explained beforehand by the worker, or preferably the worker can provide an introduction to a safe 'corner' from which the new resident can observe and learn these rules. There are other, more subtle, norms or conventions in the groups, which are sometimes harder to identify. The kind of things that can be discussed, the kind of attitudes that are acceptable to the group, etc., take some time to learn and may be slowly altered by interaction with new members.

The group situation provides residents with opportunities to explore new roles and relationships. In this sense groups can be a very positive influence. If an elderly person has lived alone, and has had few contacts for some time, he may be able to find a renewed status and sense of personal value in a group with his peers. Older people have many experiences in common in both general and more specific terms. A lifetime in the same community is bound to give common interests on which to base an initial conversation from which a closer relationship may grow. An important task for the residential worker will be to take part in the informal groupings in the home to encourage and guide the development of relationships. It will also be important to look out for those who feel left out of group interaction: by offering these people some special interest and a personal relationship it may be possible to draw them into closer relationships with the group. The individual resident will need to feel that he has an identifiable role to play in the institutional group and that the group as a whole accepts him. The worker can help to foster acceptance by example and occasionally by interpretation of difficult behaviour to the group. Painful problems can sometimes arise for group members whose self-image does not tally with the image that the group has of them.

The problems that can arise for individuals in care often tend to be emphasised by group living. At times of distress it is hard to find a quiet corner to escape to, and difficulties become exaggerated. The bad eating habits of neighbours, the mannerisms of others in the lounge, the cheerful approaches of staff can all become unbearable from time to time. Perhaps the best solution at times like these for some residents is to allow them an escape for a little while; for others the answer may be more variety, new ideas, and new activities; all residents need a personal life-space, or space to move. Flexibility of approach should again be the objective.

Sometimes resident groups treat one member of the group as a scapegoat. This is in some ways a method of achieving a greater degree of group cohesion and solidarity. If the group can come together in opposition to a common 'enemy' then this is likely to give them a feeling of strength as a group. Although this may have some positive value for those who are within the group it often creates intolerable problems for the person who is scapegoated. Sometimes this is a new member who may be seen as a threat to an existing situation and therefore rejected. The likelihood of change will provoke anxiety and the reaction will be a closing of ranks against the threat. One answer to this is the one that has already been given of smoothing the entry of new members. Another, wider answer will be to introduce a more positive view of the possibilities for new involvement. If the resident group is encouraged to rearrange itself in a wider range of different groupings then each resident will have the chance to choose several groups in which to form different relationships. If residents are less heavily invested in a single group they will be less likely to view other residents as a threat.

It is inevitable that interpersonal conflicts will arise within the group; it is also possible that conflict will arise between different groups of residents, or between residents and members of staff. The residential worker has some methods of dealing with these open to him. He may, in fact, stimulate some conflicts—about practical improvements in the home, for example—in order to produce ideas for development and positive change: conflict may have a creative function. In more bitter, destructive situations, the worker can be involved in clarifying what is really being said and making sure that both parties to the argument have understood what it is about. He can also let each party to the conflict know that he (the worker) can understand their point of view without being seen to take sides and he can help to present each to the other in a more favourable light. Every opportunity should be taken to reduce ill-feeling in a sensitive way that does not push the participants towards more entrenched positions.

Using the group situation

The residential worker is in continuous daily contact with the elderly residents and will interact with them in all kinds of different ways. The main objective of the worker is to be concerned with making the life of each individual resident as contented as possible. This will require the ability to balance needs and demands within the group to ensure that one resident does not benefit to the detriment of all the others. The major tasks will, therefore, be concerned with taking care of individual needs, but it is also possible to think about the values of providing group satisfactions.

In comparison to work with groups of younger people very little has been done with older people in groups. It seems that this has been very largely a result of mobility difficulties (physically bringing older people together in a group) and because of beliefs that older people are less able to use group experiences because of sensory deprivation. Some positive values are plain: groups of older people can provide each other with support, status, relationships, mutual interests, solidarity, group activities, etc. Perhaps the starting point for building growth experiences into the resident group should be the achievement of some degree of group cohesion. It is not enough to bring older people together in a room and suggest they have a discussion. Some starting point is necessary to provide initial stimulus. A group can best grow from its point of mutual contact or common ground: older people in care usually have local, community interests in common and the worker should identify these and build on them. It will probably also be necessary to identify a concrete goal or task for the group to start it in the right direction. Only when the group has achieved a degree of cohesion can it begin to cope with useful tasks.

One valuable area for growth and stimulation at any age is in play. For the child, play fulfils certain psychological needs: exploration, movement and activity encourage learning and growth; through play and imitation the child can explore and experiment with social roles and learn how it feels for others to be who they are; play also fulfils an important role in make-believe, or fantasy. In playing alternative roles the child or adult can find new satisfactions and alternative compensations. Play can fulfil similar functions for the elderly person. The use of music and movement sessions, whilst not acceptable to all residents provides some physical exercise, and singing stimulates the memory as well as providing the additional satisfactions of music itself and of group activity. Other kinds of leisure activities—gardening, hobbies, handicrafts—should all be possible and available for those who wish to be involved in them. Physical activity can best be maintained through play and leisure pursuits, which have the added benefit of emotional satisfactions.

In the resident group as a whole the outside world can take on an appearance of unreality. If residents are very cut off from the outside there may be a tendency to cope with the pains of isolation by pretending that nothing outside the home exists. This may account for exaggerated reactions to letters from outside, or excessive anxiety about visitors and obsessive reactions to lateness of arrival, etc. a link with the outside world may be a painful reminder of all the residents are missing. The way to avoid this is to encourage much more active family and community links. The local community can be brought in on many formal activities—coffee mornings, fund-raising, concerts, etc.—which may lead to more informal contacts. If neighbours and other local residents feel free to call in at any time this will offer a wider range of relationships and choice to residents. The reverse is also true: residents should be able to get out to the local shops, church and clubs. Some will be able to go alone, others may need to be organised into group outings, but all should be encouraged to remain in touch with the reality of the outside world. Relatives should also be encouraged to take an active part in caring for their elderly parents. Sometimes relatives feel guilty about being unable to care and may see a suggestion that they should come into the residential home to help as an accusation. Occasionally they project their guilt and become very hostile towards residential workers. Nevertheless if they can be involved they provide useful additional contacts and stimulation for residents.

Some boundaries must be set on groups: members need to be sure of how far they can go. Too much intimacy in the group can be as frightening as too little interaction, and residents will feel safer with clear boundaries and limitations. These limitations should not collude with the tendency to resist changes, nor should they be imposed in an authoritarian way. Authoritarianism is likely to force the residents into childlike roles, with all the negative connotations that that implies.

In using the group the residential worker should participate and guide individuals in their relationships, giving personal support to those who need encouragement to come further into the group. He should offer a flexible acceptance of individual and group needs but remain sufficiently apart and separate from the group to be able to preserve his personal identity. He should also be able to provide safe limits for the group and to protect individuals from group pressures.

Communication, observation, interpretation and recording

In order to carry out these tasks the worker should be able to communicate with residents, singly and in groups, and observe behaviour in order to make an assessment of need. Communication should also be a return process from worker to resident: clear information services are an essential part of the relationship between worker and older person and his family. Communication is a particular problem with the elderly, and especially those older people who are in long-term care. It is hard to find an adequate definition of communication but it seems to imply a two-way process that takes place between individuals and involves perception of a series of cues. It is important not to confuse listening to spoken words with understanding or communication. Communication is a much wider concept than simply picking up verbal messages. Information about individuals is received from many cues, static and dynamic. The kind of clothes a person wears, the way he uses facial expressions, the attitudes (physical and emotional) that he takes, information received about him from other sources, all go towards building up a picture of his short-term mood and his more lasting traits.

Communication capacities in the elderly are likely to have declined, sometimes because of disuse—losing the habit of communicating is a common problem—but more commonly because of sensory deterioration. The whole process of reacting, comprehending, focusing attention and concentrating on messages is likely to show some slowing down and this is likely to be aggravated by some degree of hearing loss, sight loss or even speech loss. Although perfect hearing may be retained until extreme old age, it is likely that some degree of high-tone hearing loss will be experienced. Deafness, of course, interferes with understanding but many older people are able to cover up their failing hearing ability for some time. Deafness is not a visible disability and is less likely to get the same understanding and acceptance that other disabilities receive. It is important to be sure that older people really have received a verbal message and are not just pretending to have understood for fear of admitting to deafness. In contrast to hearing loss, failing eyesight is much more readily recognised by the ageing person. Nevertheless many older people have inadequate aids to sight and are likely to miss the non-verbal content of communications, particularly facial expression. Speech loss is an additional complication for some older people, particular difficulties being the frustration that results for the old person and the danger that they will be assumed to be unable to understand the speech of others.

There are some essential points to be remembered about communication. It is important to give warning of communication to a deaf or blind person: they must know in advance that a message is coming or they may miss the beginning. Blind people, especially, rely on an introductory comment to be sure of whom they are talking to. Similarly it is vital to take enough time to get the message across. Older people must be allowed to receive information at their own pace. This does not just apply to those with sensory impairment: all older people should be allowed to set the pace. It is also more likely that older people will experience silences: the worker should not be made anxious by silence and rush to fill a gap in the conversation. Given time the elderly person can express himself. Another aspect of facilitating communication is the need to provide an environment in which elderly residents feel secure enough to express themselves. There may also be a feeling that there is a language, educational, culture and generational gap which must be bridged and the residential worker will have to spend time discovering and building a common basis of language with the residents. Sometimes physical touch is a useful part of establishing a communication link.

Most important of all is the provision of aids to communication, especially hearing aids and spectacles. Artificial aids to replace sensory loss can make a vast difference to levels of communication and to satisfactions.

If he is to receive communications appropriately the residential worker should also have skills in observation. The assessment and interpretation of facts that are observed will be closely related to the setting in which they take place. Behaviour that is appropriate in some situations is not appropriate to others. The cultural background, the group context, the physical environment, the aims and goals of the group, all contribute to giving meaning to the behaviour.

Referring to the earlier discussion of individual need, the worker should be able to gather information about the strengths and needs of each individual. He will also need to gather facts about how roles are allocated in the groups and how relationship patterns help or hinder individual development. The pattern of group controls on residents and the ways in which conflict and interpersonal and inter-group conflicts manifest themselves must be observed and assessed. The worker must also be aware of the state of morale in the home and of the nature and patterns of communication. In order to provide effectively for the contentment of all the residents the residential worker should be aware of facts and data about them, but only in so far as those facts are relevant to meeting the total group needs (balancing competing demands) and in so far as they are relevant to identifying individual difficulties. Observation should not be pushed as far as intrusion into privacy.

One valuable tool in making an assessment is the use of recorded written material. This may be material relating to individuals and also to total group developments. Ongoing records serve the purpose of helping the worker to clarify the relevance of information and the nature of difficult areas, and they help in planning clearly for the future. As far as the individual resident is concerned a record of his progress will contain an implicit recognition of his right to a process of life. Life in a home or hospital should not be static: it should contain opportunities for change and extension of activities and these opportunities should have a planned rationale which will be aided and clarified by recording of development.

Other important elements in planning care are associated with the need for regular re-evaluation. Progress should be monitored by regular review procedures which facilitate an ongoing assessment. Review may be by the residential workers or by a group of professionals involved with the residents, taking the form of a case conference in the hospital. It is important that older people are not dumped in institutions and forgotten: a regular check should be kept on their needs and development.

An integrated strategy for institutional intervention

In the smaller group situation that is likely to occur in an old people's home change may be relatively easy. It is plain from the available evidence that this is not always the case, and in the larger hospital group change is likely to be a very slow process. Many structural and interpersonal constraints exist to slow down or stop change. Any strategy aimed at making a home or hospital a better place to live in should take account of all the varying factors that exist within the social system and should set out to approach change on several levels.

Self-help and participation

A geriatric hospital might be described as having three major tasks in relation to individuals: any or all of these may be carried out at any one time.
1 The primary task of the hospital is the treatment of illness or disease, with the object of returning the elderly person to his own home.
2 Some patients cannot return home, usually because of a com-

bination of disability and inadequate social supports; very few long-stay patients require other than good nursing and rehabilitative care. For these patients the therapeutic objective is one of limited rehabilitation: to improve capacities for self-care to the maximum level.

3 In a long-stay situation a further task will be concerned with providing a healthy and stimulating social environment. The long-stay ward will be a place in which some people will live for several years and it must offer a satisfying quality of life.

Residential care is less concerned with treatment (although it might be argued that if hospitals can offer medical treatment then residential homes can offer social treatment and rehabilitation) but residential workers will certainly be involved in the maintenance and improvement of levels of self-care and with the creation of a good living environment. The usual way of achieving the second of these objectives—the improvement and maintenance of self-care—has been by direct intervention with the individual. Patients are encouraged by nursing staff, occupational therapists, physiotherapists, etc., to do things for themselves: normally this means encouraging them to dress, go to the toilet, bath and feed themselves alone, and to experiment with simple home-care tasks, such as making a cup of tea, preparing a hot drink or making up a bed. The problems of this approach are mainly associated with lack of staffing resources, which results in insufficient time being available for individual patients. It is much easier and quicker to help an old man to put on his shirt than to stand back and encourage him to do it by himself. A further problem is that patients are likely to become distressed, or aggressive and abusive towards staff, if they cannot understand the underlying objective. A common patient reaction is to insist that nurses are paid to care for them and should allow patients to be dependent. This naturally puts pressure and strain on the nurse or residential worker, and for untrained staff this is particularly hard to withstand. A lot of good work can also be undone by ancillary staff who find it hard to watch older people struggle and rush to help them.

An essentially behaviourist approach of reward and punishment for successful efforts at self-care is a time-consuming and often stressful process for caring staff. It is particularly fruitless if the older person has nothing to look forward to in his day other than sitting in a day room staring at the wall or the television. It has been suggested earlier that a range of roles and relationships will offer choice and decision-making opportunities to the older patient or resident. If choice can be extended and the range of available interaction increased this will offer more interesting stimulation to the older person. If he has something to look forward to in his day, and particularly something that offers variety from day to day, then this may offer him an increased motivation to improve his capacity for self-care. A contented person who is interested in what is going on around him is more likely to want to get up and dressed in a morning.

In other words self-care capacities can be improved by beginning with the individual and encouraging him to face the environment and also increasing individual motivation more indirectly. Self-help can be viewed in this individual sense of patients being able to help themselves with daily living tasks but it may also be defined in rather wider terms as the ability to take part in the kind of care that is being offered. Elderly patients and residents have a right to be involved in decisions that are being made about what is to be done to, and for, them. They should be able to participate in the decision-making process of the institution, as well as in decisions about individual care. Of course, many will be too mentally or physically infirm to cope with this kind of involvement but others can offer very valuable contributions and increase their personal self-esteem in the process.

Older people can be encouraged to become a more significant part of the whole community through participation in staff meetings. It is likely that patients will need a lot of support and encouragement in this kind of expectation: it will demand that they adopt a new role in relation to caring staff and this will need a period of adjustment. They may also be able to control more of their lives by forming groups or committees with specific objectives: fund-raising to buy a colour television, or a mini-bus for outings, is a very cohesive and stimulating force. Once again the period of adjustment to this new kind of group may be a difficult one.

Residents, and more especially patients, may react with hostility to an initial suggestion that they should take part in a patients' committee, or in a staff group. This may be related to two factors. In the first place older people in institutions have an expectation that they will be dependent on staff: a suggestion that they can act for themselves, or give advice to staff, is a complete reversal of this expectation and will present a threat and consequent anxieties. In the second place putting patients or residents in a group and throwing them on to their own resources can be threatening and confusing without clear goals and objectives. An initial stimulus and direction will have to come from members of the staff to give cohesion through the presentation of a concrete task. Unfortunately the initial stimulus may slip into directiveness and a balance must be found between encouragement and paternalism. Although fund-raising committees are probably of most benefit to the few older people who are actually members, they do contribute to the general spirit of respect for patients and residents and encourage new activities. Participation in groups offers opportunities to increase self-esteem and status through role exploration, especially leadership roles.

Intervention and the organisation

The hospital, and to a lesser extent the residential home, offers a number of advantages and disadvantages to bringing about change. The advantages are related in particular to the possibilities of extending educational input in professional groupings: increasing knowledge may facilitate change. Disadvantages are linked to the pains of the tasks that have to be carried out which lead to highly formalised patterns of response. Topliss (1974) has described the value of communication procedures in facilitating adaptation to changing hospital goals but emphasises the risk of a good hospital communication system being allowed to atrophy. Without the regular opportunities afforded by the communication system to re-emphasise the priorities of care the staff may tend to resort to routine if goals are general or ambiguous.

If new approaches to patient care, such as increasing patient participation, are developed the objectives must be clearly discussed with all members of staff. An emphasis on patient participation and self-care is likely to increase the demands, both physical and emotional, that are made on staff. This is especially true of staff who are in continual contact with patients or residents—nurses and residential workers. An attempt to affect organisational goals and established patterns of behaviour must also include increased staff-support groups.

Community and family links

Some of the values of encouraging the links of people within the institutional group have already been examined. An intervention strategy that is confined solely to the world inside the institution will deal with an unreal perspective. Community resources can be used in many ways to bring in new ideas and stimuli: the hospital or home should be a part of its local community. Relatives of patients and residents can also be involved in many ways, from actually participating in providing the care (Pain, 1973), to involvement in planning for care, and to participating in discussion and support groups. Relatives can experience a good deal of relief of feeling (of guilt, anxiety, over-protection, etc.) through discussion with others and can offer mutual support and this can sometimes reduce their emotional demands on staff, residents and patients.

Working with the individual in the communal group

Relationships between professional groups

One of the results of attempting to change goals and attitudes in an institutional context is that it will involve a change in the existing pattern of relationships between different staff groupings. This will probably be more of a problem in the larger, hospital setting where many groups of professionals and ancillary staff are involved in caring. Difficulties may tend to focus themselves on issues of rigidly defining roles and responsibilities to provide a feeling of security. It may be difficult to decide whose role it is to stimulate change in particular areas of the organisation: e.g. Should the occupational therapist or the social worker run groups for patients? How far should the nurse act as the agent of other professional groups in the course of daily interaction with patients?

The answer to these difficulties seems to lie in improved communication, increased use of staff support groups, and an integrated strategy for the whole institution. In the strategy all staff members will have a recognisable and recognised role to play and they should be able to work towards an understanding, and probably a modification, of the strategy in discussion groups. Continuing education, and training exercises, will also play a very important part. Change is a slow process but if it is to take place it will require the involvement of all staff. It is not necessarily essential that all staff approve of new ideas: conflict does promote learning, new thinking, and activity. Some conflict can be a useful stimulus to realistic change, but should not be allowed to get out of hand: development comes from the resolution not the institutionalisation of conflict.

Specialist facilities in the home or hospital

As part of the need for a flexibility of approach to individuals in care it will be important to include a range of special facilities in the provision that exists. On the one hand this will require the provision of facilities for individual residents of a home to make a cup of tea for themselves and visitors, to choose library books, to buy small personal luxuries, to do small items of washing and ironing, etc. These are basic necessities of personal respect and although using a kettle or an iron may involve some risk this is an element of risk that can be taken with many residents.

Attention to physical health and appearance is another important part of provision for a contented life. Visits from optician, dentist, chiropodist, physiotherapist, etc., are very important, as is regular medical attendance. A hairdresser, for men as well as women, can also improve morale. Regular outings to the shops are a much more attractive prospect for many older residents than having a limited choice brought to the home. If residents cannot get out of the home then as much choice as possible should be brought in to them from the shops: this is especially true of clothing.

Confusion: integration or segregation

It might be thought that many of the approaches to individual need that have been described in this chapter imply a degree of rationality in the elderly resident or patient. An increasing number of elderly residents do seem to display symptoms of confusion and there is scope for considerable discussion of the appropriate style of care for the confused elderly. Whatever the institutional environment in which they are placed all elderly people are entitled to respect: the fundamental tenet of concern for the individual stands in all situations.

Meacher (1972) has argued that there are several theoretical accounts for the causation of confusion and in his discussion he emphasises the crucial role of social factors. He defines 'confusion' as displaying to a marked degree one or more of a number of characteristics, including incoherence or tangential ways of speaking, physical restlessness, disorientation of place, or the unconventional use of objects or bizarre reiteration. On the basis of this definition he studied residents in separatist and 'ordinary' homes and found a sizeable minority of confused residents in ordinary homes. He also found that separatist homes had a large minority of residents who showed no evidence of confusion and that the confused in separatist homes were less integrated into the life of the homes (perhaps a reflection of their extreme confusion on admission). Meacher goes on to suggest that some older people are 'taken for a ride' in a strange car or ambulance with inadequate explanation or clarification of where they are going. In these circumstances it is not surprising that, when asked if they know where they are, what day it is, etc., they respond in a negative, apparently disorientated way. They are therefore quite likely to be labelled as confused, especially in a separatist home, and to be treated as a confused person. If they are treated in this way the easiest response is to accept the role and play into the expectations.

Meacher argues further that separatism produces other undesirable effects on members of staff. Separating some older people may carry with it an underlying assumption or stereotype—that there is something amiss with them and they are somehow less than human. As a result special procedures and attitudes may develop in separatist homes: ritualisations (such as physical searches instead of asking), infantilising practices and belittling reproofs may occur. Staff tend to emphasise aspects of personality inadequacies rather than look to environmental deficiencies.

Bergman (1973) in a letter responding to Meacher's arguments suggests that his findings are indicative of bad environments which are not tailored to the needs of the 'confused'. He argues that (p. 595).

> a good environment would imply better and more skilled staff; more privacy, in which episodic behavioural disturbance could be tolerated; a safe, planned environment, in which restraint need only be minimally invoked; and placement of residents near to the community, to encourage friends and local voluntary workers to visit frequently.

Several studies (McKeown and Cross, 1969; Kidd, 1962; Mezey, Hodkinson and Evans, 1968) have shown that some elderly people are in the wrong place. Andrews (1972) proposes an alternative categorisation of patients with mental illness: a group with behaviour disturbance who need residential accommodation and sheltered housing mainly because of physical concomitants of ageing; a group presenting social difficulties because of forgetfulness, tiresomeness and gentle wanderings, and requiring local authority hostels for the mentally infirm; a group requiring hospital care in a geriatric department because of acute or chronic physical illness, disability, or general frailty; and finally a group requiring admission to a psychiatric hospital because of functional psychoses or neuroses needing psychiatric treatment and those needing control or tolerance not available in a general nursing context. Andrews suggests that some patients are misplaced, especially in the last two categories of geriatric and psycho-geriatric beds and that many of them can receive the care that they need equally well in either type of bed, providing local standards are adequate.

This, then is the range of the debate. There seems no doubt that some older people with forms of mental disturbance are in the wrong kind of accommodation. This seems to be important in so far as staff attitudes to 'confused behaviour' are affected and in so far as those attitudes affect the patient or resident. Social factors and expectations have an effect on the behaviour of older people and may contribute to confused behavioural manifestations. The important message to draw from the debate is perhaps that good care for the mentally infirm elderly rests on the same individual flexible resident-centred, concerned approach as care for other elderly people, whether provided in a separatist or integrated establishment.

Chapter six

Conclusions

The residential worker

So far the discussion has been focused on the needs of the elderly
resident but residential workers, too, have needs of their own: they
are also involved in a large number of practical tasks in the provision
of care, which should be considered.

The most important of these practical tasks will relate to basic
needs for food, warmth, and physical comfort. An adequate, varied
and balanced diet is essential to the older person and the provision
of food is an important element in the creating and sustaining of
relationships. Similarly, the provision of clothing and washing and
laundry facilities is a necessary contribution to individual well-being
and consequently to the relationships between worker and residents.
In the hospital setting especially, more personal demands will be
made in terms of giving medicines, bathing and dressing: much of
the most effective communication between older person and worker
may take place in the bathroom. The increasing physical dependence
of many residents is another very important factor in determining
the ways in which staff time is spent. If residents are very infirm
more time will be spent on giving essential help with daily living
needs.

The administration of practical provisions is a very large part of
the residential worker's task and the amount of support that he
receives in carrying out this function will determine the amount of
time that he has available for tasks such as promoting group
interaction and planning for individual needs. This support will take
two principal forms: the actual number of staff available to provide
care for the resident group, and the nature of staff supervision and
development, and management back-up facilities. In 1965 the
Williams Committee found there was an average of 6·3 residents to

Conclusions

each member of staff in old people's homes (Williams Report, 1967). This report suggested that an increase in the ratio of residents to staff, over a ten-year period, to 4·3:1 would require almost double the number of staff employed at the time. Even to increase the ratio to 5·3:1 would require an increase of 50 per cent in staffing over ten years. Carstairs and Morrison (1971) found that in homes in Scotland in 1969 the ratio was 6·1:1. The very large and very small homes had low ratios, a very high proportion of the smaller homes having the lowest ratio of 2·3 or fewer residents to one member of staff.

It is difficult to draw any conclusions about the need for change in staffing ratios. The needs of residents in all forms of institutional care vary considerably from the relatively fit and ambulant to the bedfast and demented. Staffing policies have to account for these variations in planning for development. In this particular area of planning and development, research into appropriate staffing levels is clearly needed.

The second major area of staff support is that of supervision and management back-up. Dealing with infirm, confused, sometimes aggressive and hostile, and frequently dependent old people is very demanding. In order to be able to separate themselves from the needs of residents and make more objective assessments workers need to be able to examine themselves and their reactions in discussion with colleagues—not necessarily administrative superiors. Within the individual old people's home or hospital ward several staff groupings are likely to be working. Nurses, doctors, occupational therapists, social workers or residential workers rely heavily on domestic staff, catering staff and other ancillary groups. All these workers are in face to face contact with patients and residents: sometimes the cleaner is likely to see as much of the old person as the residential worker. It is important that the general objectives and aims of the workers can be shared and discussed, even though information about individual residents' needs is not shared in detail. The therapeutic environment and the general living environment are bound to work more effectively if the general aims of all the workers who are involved are held in common.

The residential worker in the home should, therefore, be involved in communicating and co-ordinating the work of all the staff groupings in a general way in so far as he has such a specific management role. He should also be involved in providing specific staff support aimed at clarifying objectives in relation to individual residents. It is through discussion that plans for development begin to emerge as ideas are formulated and feelings are clarified. A similar process of support should be available for the residential worker from a management structure which can co-ordinate policy as well as offer efficient administration of resources and a channel for feeding ideas up to the agency's policy makers.

There are, of course, areas of stress for the residential worker which relate more to the conditions of working than to the fear of involvement in interpersonal relationships that lead to ritualisation and standardisation of task performance and the avoidance of decision-making. The work-situation-related problems are mainly associated with the physical demands of the task and the difficulties of escaping. Many residential workers with the elderly live actually on the premises, although difficulties of recruitment are forcing some authorities to review the general policy of living-in. The residential worker may often feel that he is on the job for twenty-four hours a day, seven days a week. In some cases this may be the literal truth because of difficulties of recruiting staff, especially night staff, or because of the nature of the living accommodation which sometimes requires workers to share facilities with residents. In these pressured circumstances it is inevitable that workers should become tired, irritable, and unable to do an effective job. Staffing policies must provide for regular breaks for residential workers, especially regular days off, and adequate annual holidays—and workers must be given the support and administrative back-up to be able to feel free to leave the home for a while.

The pressures exist whether workers are married or single, although the nature of the pressures perhaps varies. The married couple living in residential accommodation will have a need to maintain a private relationship that is separate from their professional lives. The single person will also need to be able to retain a sense of separateness by maintaining an existence outside the home.

Education, training and research

Training is a vital element in the development and use of residential workers, and one to which workers in post have an essential contribution to make. Pettes (1967) suggested that the student supervisor in social work has a threefold role as administrator, educator and helper. Ainsworth and Bridgford (1971) have developed this approach in relation to residential work. They suggest that all these must be carried out in residential work with the additional factor that the supervisor must also carry out these procedures in relation to the residents who have to take the student into their home. In the relationship between field social work student and supervisor focus is on the individual relationship between student and supervisor and on the development of the casework relationship with the client, which is essentially outside the mainstream of the client's life experience. Ainsworth and Bridgford suggest that in the residential situation 'residents, student and supervisor are sharing a primary life experience'. The residential work supervisor has not just the student's perceptions but also his own perceptions of the interaction. The period of adjustment to this wider life-space situation may cause extra tensions and anxieties for the student, which the supervisor must be prepared to give help with. Other significant differences are that the student is usually in an obvious student role in relation to residents, and that the nature of recording is likely to be aimed at day-to-day group interaction rather than at individual relationships.

It is also important for the student to be given clear boundaries to the life-space setting to provide security in involvement with the resident group. The ability to function as a member of the team, and an awareness of group process, are also valuable aspects of training. Mattinson (1968) suggests the area to be covered in supervision should be: techniques in handling residents; individual pathology; resident interaction; staff interaction; methods of management, case- and problem-centred; use of self and own strengths in this situation, group- and student-centred; discussion of the process of interaction in the whole community. Ainsworth and Bridgford propose six differences in the contexts of field and residential work supervision: residential work supervision is concerned with the social system rather than the dyadic approach; it is concerned with the life-space rather than the interview situation; the resident is aware of the student role; the supervisor in residential care is involved in primary interaction with residents; the student is involved in primary experience rather than associate experience as in the casework relationship; recording in residential work is likely to be in diary form rather than process recording.

A research report carried out on behalf of the Central Council for Education and Training in Social Work (Curnock, 1975) has shown how little use is made of residential experience in student placements. Much more use could be made of residential placements not simply as short-term observation experience but as fully developed placements on an equal basis with placements in other settings. It does appear that if training in residential work is to be extended then new techniques of supervision and evaluation may have to be developed. Training for residential work with the elderly will require special emphasis on the particular needs of older people, especially involving an understanding of their physical needs.

The problem of education and attitudes to working with the elderly is a much wider one than simply extending the skills of field and residential workers and doctors and paramedical workers. The ways in which institutions are used to provide care and the expectations and attitudes that are held towards the elderly are a problem of our wider society. There is a need for education at all levels on how to use old age and how to live a satisfactory life after retirement. If old age can be seen in less stereotyped ways and older people can learn to expect change in their lives then residential facilities can begin to be used in less static ways.

Research in relation to the elderly in care is also an area that needs development. Research has concentrated on community needs of older people but, on the whole, has neglected the residential setting. There is still a common assumption that when old people go into a home they cease to have a significant existence. Research aimed at establishing the nature of continuing needs for care within homes, especially with regard to staffing needs, may encourage new developments.

Providing care for the elderly in long-term situations makes special demands on residential staff. Training which gives basic information about the social, physiological and emotional needs of older people, as well as an understanding of the communal group needs—the life-space situation—is an essential prerequisite to an improved use of residential care. Another important prerequisite is for a review of attitudes to the elderly and education in wider terms to encourage a more flexible, fluid use of institutions in a community context. The residential worker must be equipped with skills in communication and observation and with knowledge of group and communal contexts. He must also be able to provide an efficient management service in making available practical resources to elderly individuals. Most important of all he must be able to achieve a balance between the needs of individual residents and a smooth efficient running of the environment in which residents have to live.

Future needs and alternatives: the continuum

It has been suggested that hospitals and old people's homes are only a part of the whole cycle, or continuum, of caring services. The great majority of older people live a continuing, satisfying life in the community and institutional care may play a minor part in their lives. For many of these people other forms of help will be more important. A lot of emphasis is now being placed on domiciliary care for the elderly. In the main this rests on services provided by local authority social services departments. The home help service is offering a developing support service to an increasing proportion of old people. A home help can provide not only practical help in cleaning, shopping, etc., but often builds up a close relationship with clients. This relationship can help to give emotional as well as practical support and the home help may have a significant role in identifying problems in the older person's life. Some older people live a fairly precarious existence only just on the right side of coping with their everyday needs but continue to manage with good support from family and friends. If something changes in the situation—the death of a friend or relative, increasing brain failure, illness, etc.—the balance may be upset. If the home help is in contact she can help by identifying the deterioration in the general situation and providing referral to the appropriate service before things have gone too far.

Other services in the community, such as meals-on-wheels, laundry services, social workers, health visitors, etc., each has an important role to play in building up a pattern of support which can maintain the older person in the community for a long time. As long as safeguards in the form of early warning systems are built into the support network most older people can be maintained in their own home. Shaw (1971) has added a warning to the emphasis on domiciliary care. He reported on several old people who were living in very deteriorated conditions in Sheffield, at a time when a policy of keeping people out of residential care wherever possible was being followed by the local authority. Shaw argues that emphasising the absolute value of domiciliary care leads to serious problems for a few older people.

A relatively recent development has been the growth of day care centres providing a range of services which a club would not normally offer. The older person visits on a daily basis, returning home at night. Up to now this kind of development has been in relation to local needs and resources and Morley (1974) suggests that 'the impact this [the growth of day care] will make on the problem of retirement and frailty has to be seen in relation to all services offered in any one area'. Day hospital facilities have also begun to develop: the day hospital offers treatment that would normally be hospital based but which does not require in-patient care. Day hospitals are distinct from day centres in that they do not have the relief of social need as a primary aim, although this may be a secondary effect. Particular difficulties of day care facilities are the problem of finding transport, of finding adequate buildings, of finance, and of returning home to cold empty houses at the end of the day. Clearly, training of workers in day centres is an important issue: the particular context requires particular skills, many of which will be similar to those of other workers with the elderly. Morley suggests ways of improving current provision of day care services: by an increase in transport facilities and staffing; by introducing additional supportive and ancillary services; by using members' skills in running and organising activities; and by a training scheme for paid and unpaid staff.

For some older people boarding-out schemes may be a suitable answer to their need for care. Some schemes have been run by voluntary agencies and by local authorities but with apparently limited success. Boarding-out may be a more suitable solution for negotiation in individual cases. The principal difficulties are likely to be ones of financial support of the old person, and matching the needs of the older person with those of the hostess. Perhaps short-term boarding has something to offer in cases of elderly people who normally live alone during the initial period after hospital discharge. It should certainly be viewed as an additional resource to be considered when planning for care.

The relationship between housing needs, need for admission to care, and depression, etc., has been recorded by several studies (see, for example, Townsend and Wedderburn, 1965). An increased use of sheltered housing schemes may improve the situation. One important implication is for the role of the warden in such schemes, which, to be most effective, cannot be restricted to offering only an emergency scheme or maintenance of the housing. At the other extreme it is equally unrealistic to expect one warden to offer personal support with self-care needs—dressing, cooking, lighting fires, shopping, etc.—for the members of fifty or more households. Effective training for wardens will recognise the need for a balance between a remote, emergency service, and an over-demanding exhausting service. The task of the warden in grouped housing, like that of the residential worker, is to find a balance between individual need and the efficient running of a service to all the tenants.

One study (Wager, 1972) has set out to examine the relative resource cost to the community of providing domiciliary or residential care. As a cost benefit analysis it aimed to include all significant costs and benefits irrespective of the authority or individual to whom they accrued: the everyday costs of living an independent life in the community were considered alongside the costs of accommodation and services provided by local authorities. Wager's comparative examination of the resource costs of domiciliary and residential care led him to conclude that (p. 65):

> for those living in sheltered housing or lower value 'normal'
> housing there was, on average, a margin of £3 or £4 per week
> to be taken up by domiciliary services before domiciliary care
> reached the cost of residential care. Having regard to the
> current levels of provision of domiciliary services, this offers a
> substantial scope for the expansion of domiciliary care.

In more expensive housing the margin tended to be smaller or negative, but there is clearly evidence here that residential care is a relatively expensive provision in economic terms. It should, of course, be remembered that inflation has affected the figures, though not the principle.

Another study (Blenkner, 1966) may throw further light on the emphasis on domiciliary care. This study set out to reduce hospital admission by providing intensive domiciliary care for an experimental group of clients. At the end of the study more of the clients in the experimental group had been admitted to the hospital than had members of the control group. It may be, in fact, that too much care in the home is as bad as too little care in that it encourages dependent behaviour patterns.

If all the available means of keeping the elderly client in the community are insufficient for his needs then residential care must be a viable alternative. A study by Simpson (1971) looked at three county council homes for the elderly in order to assess the effects of differences in design and staffing roles on residential care, as measured especially by residents' daily activities. The first home was a two-year old home in which residents lived in self-contained flats, each for eight residents. The staff played a 'supportive' role rather than 'caring for' residents, who were left to do much of their own cooking and cleaning. The second of the homes was four years old, with four sitting rooms, one large dining room and kitchen and long corridors of bedrooms. Staff generally did more for the residents and although daily household activities could be carried out there were fewer facilities for doing so. The third home was much older and was partly converted from an old house: there were no private kitchens, dining room or utility room. Although the design was much like that of the second home one of the three sitting rooms was very large, with chairs lined up around the walls. Residents were used to most things being done by staff and they were not encouraged to do any housework themselves.

There were several significant conclusions to the study. The death rate in the oldest home was higher than in any of the other homes. On the basis of staff assessment the residents in the first home were more mobile than those in the second, who were more mobile that those in the third; the first home also had the greatest amount of physical activity. A similar ranking order was found for those residents who did housework, who used the kitchen and who talked more often. The residents of the first home were also less likely to be doing nothing, less likely to be reading and less likely to attend church services and clubs. The main suggestions of the study are that the first home, where personal independence is possible because of design factors and because it is encouraged by staff, shows the greatest degree of overall physical activity and of social activity.

It seems safe to assume from this evidence that it is a mistake to lump 'residential accommodation' together in a single entity.

Different influences are at work, and two of these are staff attitudes and practices and the physical design of the home. Not only must community resources be flexibly used but the differences in residential care must be identified and built into individual treatment programmes.

Social rehabilitation and residential care

Several references have already been made to the therapeutic element in residential care in relation to an overall plan for social treatment in a community context. Some older people do deteriorate because of a combination of factors but following admission to care begin to thrive. Although the actual numbers of such people are few at the moment this may reflect current use of residential resources rather than the potential uses. The old people's homes and the hospital, whether acute or longstay, are a part of the community and their potential use as a treatment resource can be seen in two particular contexts. In one relatively undeveloped sense residential care could be used in much more flexible ways—to extend the current practice of giving holiday relief to relatives, to take older people during the winter months or while the family move house or decorate the house. Perhaps one possibility is admission for a few months as a deliberate treatment method to use the factors that exist in the enclosed communal situation to improve the elderly client's capacity to cope alone.

The more usual method of using residential care is admission to overcome environmental or emotional stress that can no longer be coped with in the client's own home. The key factor in this situation is the recognition of the older person's need to return to a process of life, and not to be treated in a stereotyped way. This implies full careful assessment of needs before, during and after admission and regular review of client needs in order to provide for changing needs and circumstances.

If this is to be a feasible proposition the field worker and residential worker will have to develop good working relationships. In building up such relationships they are likely to meet a number of special difficulties. If it is true, for instance, that the institution builds up an internal defence system then the field worker, who presents the painful reality of the outside world, may present a threat to the defence system. The conflict of the field worker, in giving up even a part of his client to the residential worker, is also likely to exist for the latter who may find difficulty in sharing the people in his care with other workers. In addition to these difficulties there may also be a real difference in the kind of context in which field worker and residential worker function. The field worker is concerned essentially with the individual client and his interpersonal relationships; the residential worker is concerned with the life-space situation in the home. In an ideal world this division should not exist: each worker is concerned with the functioning of the individual elderly person and the social system in which he is living at any one point in time. In the real world there is a physical division between the home and the outside world and workers will perceive a difference in context, which is very likely to include differences in attitudes, language, status, etc.

It is extremely important that these differences are resolved and that good working relationships are built up. Communication is very necessary for both workers to get a complete picture of the elderly individual and for them to be able to deal with the whole person. Incomplete communication leads to dealing in stereotypes, abbreviations and labelling. The danger of labelling residents and consequently failing to deal with a complete person is quite considerable and may result from a careless conversation before admission. Positive labels can be as damaging as negative ones in so far as they may also prevent the worker relating to the whole person. Full information should be shared between residential worker and field worker at admission to overcome this problem.

A good relationship between workers is also essential to facilitate the process of admission (and discharge) for the patient or resident and to facilitate ongoing contact between field worker and client. The elderly client should not just be taken to the home and abandoned by the field worker, thus emphasising the total rejection of society. Even if he only visits two or three times it is important for the field worker to acknowledge the continuing existence of the client and spend some time in handing over the client to the residential worker. It is important to maintain the continuing contact for some older people to present them with wider opportunities for extending roles out into the community wherever possible.

A further reason for the continued contact between field and residential worker is the need for professional exchange and mutual support. It is mainly by informal contacts that each learns of the needs, attitudes and expectations of the other. If a good relationship can be established then residential accommodation can be used more flexibly and sensitively to meet individual needs.

Final summary

In working with the elderly in residential accommodation, and to a large extent in long-stay hospitals, two factors are central:

(1) Ageing is a process, or rather a collection of processes, and it

is a process in which we are all involved. Social and health services have all too often been based on stereotyped assumptions about old age. 'Old age' as a static, stereotyped grouping does not exist: certainly there is a growing number of people who are older than retirement age but the needs that older people present are as widely diffuse as the needs of any age grouping. For the great majority of people growing old is a process of becoming less involved in wider social roles associated particularly with employment situations. Contrary to some assumptions this withdrawal from wide social roles does not involve withdrawal from family and friendship ties. Most people are quite closely tied into their community and family networks by the services they receive and provide for others. For a minority of old people the ageing process may lead them to encounter a number of characteristic problems. Most people do manage to cope with these problems but some older people suffer from the combined effects of interrelated difficulties with which they are unable to cope alone. For these people there are a range of caring services available to meet the needs.

(2) Residential care is one part of this range of services. Although there are many alternatives to residential care that can be provided in the community—home helps, meals on wheels, voluntary help, day centres, day hospitals, lunch clubs, etc.—residential care or hospital care may be the best answer for some people, either for a temporary or a long-term period.

In using institutional situations to the best advantage it is important to be aware of the way the internal social system of the institution can build up routines and make its own demands on those who have to live within it. Problems of admission stress, and of the attitudes of old people to themselves and to those who provide care, as well as the attitudes of others to the older people, can also create problems for the flexible use of caring resources.

The residential worker is concerned with easing the new resident into the communal group and with supporting him while he recovers from the crisis he has been through. He is also concerned with creating a contented, ongoing process of life for all the residents by the flexible use of individual relationships, of group interaction and of the total life-space situation. Perhaps most important of all the residential worker must recognise the fact that no individual's needs will remain static: the residential environment must provide for change in group and individual needs. The worker should seek to find a balance between individual needs and the efficient running of the institution.

Successful care, in any situation, for the older person in need will involve a recognition that solutions should aim to deal not just with a limited view of the here-to-now but should be concerned with the

Conclusions

restoration of an ageing process, with the satisfactions that this will imply. The individual ageing process can continue with satisfactions and contentment in residential care if workers recognise the need to seek a pattern of successful ageing for each individual in a flexible way.

Suggestions for further reading

Although the literature relating specifically to ageing is increasing quite rapidly, much of it relates mainly to American society and very little of it is aimed directly at institutional care. The problem for the worker is therefore one of identifying material from many sources and bringing it together with some relevance to residential work practice. In a slightly different, but related, context I have drawn together some of the literature with regard to field social work practice (*Social Work, Ageing and Society*, 1975) and this may provide a useful starting point for additional reading.

The literature on institutions is quite extensive: some of the significant works have been mentioned in the text (see chapter 2). Useful general books are those by Goffman (*Asylums*, 1961), Miller and Gwynne (*A Life Apart*, 1972), and King, Raynes and Tizard (*Patterns of Residential Care*, 1971). Three important books that give insight into what happens to older people in institutions are the works of Townsend (*The Last Refuge*, 1962), Meacher (*Taken for a Ride*, 1972), and Robb (*Sans Everything*, 1967). The reports of the Ely (1969), Farleigh (1971) and Whittingham (1972) Committees of Inquiry are also valuable reading.

There are several basic books dealing with specific aspects of ageing. Especially helpful is *The Psychology of Human Ageing* (Bromley, 1974), and a book edited by Chown (*Human Ageing*, 1972a) is also helpful on psychological aspects of ageing. Blau (*Old Age in a Changing Society*, 1973) gives a wide range of ideas on the sociological aspects of ageing. The cross-national study of old people in industrial society by Shanas et al. (*Old People in Three Industrial Societies*, 1968) is a very thorough study of the social, family and occupational needs of the elderly. The related study of loneliness and isolation by Tunstall (*Old and Alone*, 1966) also provides good basic ideas. On physical and psychiatric changes useful starting

101

points will be found in books by Whitehead (*Psychiatric Disorders in Old Age*, 1974) and by Agate (*Geriatrics for Nurses and Social Workers*, 1972).

An increasing amount of straightforward and basic literature is being provided by Age Concern, the national voluntary organisation and much of this is relevant to special needs and provisions. Other books dealing with special needs are by Felstein (*Sex in Later Life*, 1973) and by Hinton (*Dying*, 1967). The latter book is a good introduction to the subject of death and dying.

One other important study of the effectiveness of social work with the elderly by Goldberg (*Helping the Aged*, 1970) is essential reading.

Bibliography

Agate, J. (1970), *The Practice of Geriatrics*, Heinemann Medical Books.
Agate, J. (1972), *Geriatrics for Nurses and Social Workers*, Heinemann Medical Books.
Age Concern (1971), *Age Concern on Pensioner Incomes*, Age Concern.
Age Concern (1974), *Training for Wardens of Grouped Housing Schemes—Report and Recommendations of Working Group*, Age Concern.
Ainsworth, F. and Bridgford, N. (1971), 'Student supervision in residential work', *Brit. J. Social Work*, vol. 1, no. 4, pp. 455-62.
Andrews, J. (1972), 'The future of the psychogeriatric patient', in *The Elderly Mind*, *Brit. Hospit. J.* and Hospital International in conjunction with the Kings Fund Centre and the British Hospital Export Council.
Barton, R. (1959), *Institutional Neurosis*, Wright.
Bates, F. L. (1956), 'Position, role and status: a reformulation of concepts', *Social Forces*, vol. 34, May.
Beattie, W. (1972), *Social Adaptation: Research Perspectives and Practice Requirements*, Proc. IXth Int. Cong. Geront., Kiev, USSR.
Belknap, I. (1956), *Human Problems of a State Mental Hospital*, McGraw-Hill.
Bennett, A. E., Deane, M., Elliott, A. and Holland, W. W. (1968), 'Care of old people in residential homes', *Brit. J. Prev. Soc. Med.*, vol. 22, pp. 193-8.
Bergman, K. (1973), letter to *New Society*, vol. 22, no. 531.
Berry, J. (1972), 'The experience of reception into residential care', *Brit. J. Social Work*, vol. 2, no. 4, pp. 423-34.
Birren, J. (1972), *The Organisation of Behaviour, Adaptation, and Control of Ageing*, Proc. IXth Int. Cong. Geront., Kiev, USSR.
Blank, M. L. (1971), 'Recent research findings on practice with the ageing', *Social Casework*, vol. 52, no. 6, pp. 382-9.
Blau, Z. S. (1973), *Old Age in a Changing Society*, New Viewpoints, Watts.
Blenkner, M. (1965), 'Social work and family relationships in later life with some thoughts on filial maturity', in E. Shanas and C. Streib (eds), *Social Structure and the Family*, Prentice-Hall.
Blenkner, M. (1966), *Environmental Change and the Ageing Individual*, Proc. VIIth Int. Cong. Geront., Vienna, Austria.
Boldy, D., Abel, P. and Carter, K. (1973), *The Elderly in Grouped Dwellings: A Profile*, Institute of Biometry and Community Medicine, publication no. 3, University of Exeter.
Booth, A. and Hess, E. (1974), 'Cross-sex friendship', *Journal of Marriage and the Family*, vol. 36, no. 1, p. 38.
Boucher, C. A. (1957), *Survey of Services Available to the Chronic Sick and Elderly in 1954-55*, Reports on Public Health and Medical Subjects, no. 98, HMSO.
Bowlby, J. (1951), *Maternal Care and Mental Health*, WHO, Geneva.
Bowlby, J. (1969), *Attachment and Loss: I.Attachment*, Hogarth Press.

103

Bibliography

Brearley, C. P. (1972), 'Waiting for age', *Social Work Today*, vol. 3, no. 18.

Brearley, C. P. (1975), *Social Work, Ageing and Society*, Routledge & Kegan Paul.

Bromley, D. B. (1974), *The Psychology of Human Ageing*, Penguin Books.

Burton, J. (1974), 'Poverty, deprivation and the crisis in social work: policy or structure', *Social Work Today*, vol. 5, no. 15.

Carstairs, V. and Morrison, M. (1971), *The Elderly in Residential Care*, Scottish Home and Health Department, Health Service Studies no. 19.

Cartwright, A., Hockey, L. and Anderson, J. L. (1973), *Life Before Death*, Routledge & Kegan Paul.

Caudill, W. (1958), *The Psychiatric Hospital as a Small Society*, Harvard University Press.

Central Council for Education and Training in Social Work (1973), *Training for Residential Work—Discussion Document*, CCETSW.

Central Council for Education and Training in Social Work (1974), *Paper 3: Residential Work is a Part of Social Work*, Report of the Working Party on Education for Residential Social Work, CCETSW.

Chown, S. M. (1972a), *Human Ageing*, Penguin Books.

Chown, S. M. (1972b), 'Psychological and emotional aspects of ageing', in *Easing the Restrictions of Ageing*, Age Concern.

Chown, S. M. and Davies, A. D. M. (1972), 'Age effects on speed and level of intelligence test performance', in S.M. Chown (1972a).

Crawford, M. (1972), 'Retirement and role-playing', *Sociology*, vol. 6, no. 2.

Cumming, E. and Henry, W. E. (1961), *Growing Old: The Process of Disengagement*, Basic Books.

Curnock, K. (1975), *Student Units in Social Work Education*, CCETSW.

Department of Health (Scotland) (1953), *The Ageing Population*, HMSO.

Dowd, J. J. (1975), 'Ageing and exchange: a preface to theory', *J. Geront.*, vol. 30, no. 5, pp. 584-94.

Ely Report (1969), *Report of the Committee of Inquiry into Allegations of Ill-treatment of Patients ... at Ely Hospital, Cardiff*, Cmnd 3975, HMSO.

Erikson, E. (1950), *Childhood and Society*, Norton.

Etzioni, A. (1960), 'Interpersonal and structural factors in the study of mental hospitals', *Psychiatry*, vol. 23, no. 1.

Farleigh Report (1971), *Report of the Farleigh Hospital Committee of Inquiry*, Cmnd 4557, HMSO.

Felstein, I. (1973), *Sex in Later Life*, Penguin Books.

Finkle, A. L. (1971), 'Sexual function during advancing age', in I. Rossman (ed.), *Clinical Geriatrics*, Lippincott.

Froimovich, J. and Acle, V. (1972), *Therapeutic Effect on the Adaptation of the Aged*, Proc. IXth Int. Cong. Geront., Kiev, USSR.

Fry, M. (1954), 'Old age looks at itself', in *Old Age in the Modern World*, Report of the 3rd Congress of the International Association of Gerontology, Livingstone.

Gilhome, K. (1974), 'Emotional needs', in *The Place of the Retired and Elderly in Modern Society—Views of Manifesto Discussion Groups*, Age Concern.

Gilmore, A. J. J. (1975), 'Some characteristics of non-surviving subjects in a 3-year longitudinal study of elderly people living at home', *Geront. Clin.*, vol. 17, pp. 72-9.

Gilmore, A. J. J. and Caird, F. I. (1972), 'Locating the elderly at home', *Age and Ageing*, vol. 1, no. 3.

Goffman, E. (1961), *Asylums: Essays on the Social Situation of Mental Patients and Other Inmates*, Doubleday.

Goldberg, E. M. (1970), *Helping the Aged*, NISWT Series, Allen & Unwin.

Goldman, R. (1971), 'Decline in organ function with ageing', in I. Rossman (ed.), *Clinical Geriatrics*, Lippincott.

Gore, I. Y. (1972), 'Physical activity and ageing—a survey of the Soviet literature', *Geront. Clin.*, vol. 14, no. 2, pp. 65-86.

Greenblatt, M., Levinson, D. J. and Williams, R. H. (eds) (1957), *The Patient and the Mental Hospital*, Collier-Macmillan.

Hall, M. R. P. (1972), 'Physical health', in *Easing the Restrictions of Ageing*, Age Concern.

Hanson, J. (1971), *Residential Care Observed*, NISWT and Age Concern.

Bibliography

Harris, A. I. (1968), *Social Welfare for the Elderly*, Government Social Survey, HMSO.

Harris, C. C. (1972), *The Deprivation Theory of Old Age: The Generic Mode*, Proc. IXth Int. Cong. Geront., Kiev, USSR, Symposia Reports, vol. 2, pp. 255-7.

Havighurst, R. J. (1968), 'Personality and patterns of ageing', *Gerontologist*, vol. 8, pp. 20-3.

Hinton, J. M. (1963), 'The physical and mental distress of the dying', *Quart. J. Med.*, N.S.32, 1.

Hinton, J. M. (1967), *Dying*, Penguin Books.

Hobman, D. (1972), 'Changing roles and relationships', in *Easing the Restrictions of Ageing*, Age Concern.

Karn, V. (1977), *Retiring to the Seaside*, Routledge & Kegan Paul.

Kay, D. W. K., Norris, V. and Post, F. (1956), 'Prognosis in psychiatric disorders of the elderly', *J. Ment. Sc.*, 102, p. 129.

Kent, E. A. (1963), 'Role of admission stress in adaptation of older persons in institutions', *Geriatrics*, February, pp. 133-8.

Kerckhoff, A. C. (1964), 'Husband and wife expectations and reactions to retirement', *J. Gerontol.* vol. 19, pp. 510-16.

Kidd, C. B. (1962), 'Misplacement of the elderly in hospital; a study of patients admitted to geriatric and mental hospitals', *Brit. Med. J.* (ii), 1491.

King, R. D., Raynes, N. V. and Tizard, J. (1971), *Patterns of Residential Care*, Routledge & Kegan Paul.

Kinsey, A. C., Pomeroy, W. B. and Martin, C. E. (1948), *Sexual Behaviour in the Human Male*, Saunders.

Klein, M. (1960), *Our Adult World and Its Roots in Infancy*, Tavistock.

Lamerton, R. (1973), *Care of the Dying*, Priory Press.

Lawton, M. P. (1970), 'Ecology and ageing', in L. A. Pastalan and D. H. Carson (eds), *The Spatial Behaviour of Older People*, Ann Arbor.

Levinson, D. J. (1959), 'Role, personality and social structure in the organisation setting', *J. Abnormal Soc. Psychol.*, vol. 58.

Liebermann, M. A. (1961), 'Relationship of mortality rates to entrance to a home for the aged', *Geriatrics*, October, pp. 515-19.

Litin, E. M. (1956), 'Mental reaction to trauma and hospitalisation in the aged', *J. Am. Med. Assoc.*, vol. 162, no. 17, pp. 1522-4.

McKeown, T. and Cross, K. W. (1969), 'Responsibilities of hospitals and local authorities for elderly patients', *Brit. J. Prev. Soc. Med.*, vol. 23, pp. 34-9.

Masters, W. H. and Johnson, V. E. (1966), *Human Sexual Response*, Little, Brown.

Mattinson, J. (1968), 'Supervising a residential student', *Case Conference*, vol. 14, no. 12, pp. 451-5.

Meacher, M. (1970), 'The old: the future of community care', in *The Fifth Social Service*, Fabian Society.

Meacher, M. (1972), *Taken for a Ride: Special Residential Homes for Confused Old People: A Study of Separatism in Social Policy*, Longman.

Menzies, I. E. P. (1960), 'A case study in the functioning of social systems as a defence against anxiety', *Hum. Relat.*, vol. 13, pp. 95-121.

Mezey, A. C., Hodkinson, H. M. and Evans, G. J. (1968), 'The elderly in the wrong unit', *Brit. Med. J.* (iii), pp. 16-18.

Miller, E. J. and Gwynne, G. V. (1972), *A Life Apart*, Tavistock.

Ministry of Health (1955), Circular 3/55, HMSO.

Ministry of Health (1957), Circular 14/57, HMSO.

Ministry of Health (1965), Circular 18/65, HMSO.

Ministry of Housing and Local Government (1957), Circular 55/57, HMSO.

Ministry of Pensions and National Insurance (1966), *Financial and Other Circumstances of Retirement Pensioners*, Report of an Enquiry by the Ministry of Pensions and National Insurance, HMSO.

Morley, D. (1974), *Day Care and Leisure Provision for the Elderly*, Age Concern.

Morris, B. (1971), 'Reflections on role analysis', *Brit. J. Sociol.*, vol. 22, pp. 395-409.

Neill, J. E., Fruin, D., Goldberg, E. M. and Warburton, R. W. (1973), 'Reactions to integration', *Social Work Today*, vol. 4, no. 15.

Pain, A. (1973), *Sharing the Care at Eastwood*, Age Concern Today, no. 7, Autumn.

Parsons, T. (1951), *The Social System*, Free Press.

Bibliography

Personal Social Services Council (1975), *Living and Working in Residential Homes*, PSSC.

Pettes, D. (1967), *Supervision in Social Work*, NISWT Series, Allen & Unwin.

Pfeiffer, E., Verwoerdt, A. and Wang, H. (1968), 'The natural history of sexual behaviour in aged men and women', *Arch. Gen. Psychiat.*, vol. 19, p. 753.

Phillips Committee (1954), *Report of the Committee on the Economic and Financial Problems of the Provision for Old Age*, Comnd 9333, HMSO.

Reichel, W. (1965), 'Complications in the care of five hundred hospitalized patients', *J. Amer. Geriatrics Soc.*, vol. 13, no. 11, pp. 973-81.

Robb, B. (1967), *Sans Everything—A Case to Answer*, Nelson.

Rosin, A. J. and Boyd, R. V. (1966), 'Complications of illness in geriatric patients in hospital', *J. Chron. Dis.*, vol. 19, pp. 307-13.

Rosow, I. (1967), *Social Integration of the Aged*, Free Press.

Rutter, M. (1972), *Maternal Deprivation Reassessed*, Penguin Books.

Salzberger-Wittenberg, I. (1970), *Psycho-Analytic Insight and Relationships: A Kleinian Approach*, Routledge & Kegan Paul.

Saunders, C. (1967), 'The management of terminal illness', *Hospital Medicine*, February, pp. 433-5.

Shanas, E. et al. (1968), *Old People in Three Industrial Societies*, Routledge & Kegan Paul.

Shaw, J. (1971), *On Our Conscience*, Penguin Books.

Sherman, S. R. (1975), 'Patterns of contacts for residents of age-segregated housing', *J. Geront.*, vol. 30, no. 1, pp. 103-7.

Simpson, A. (1971), *The Success of Home Close: A New Design in Residential Care for the Elderly*, Cambridgeshire and Isle of Ely County Council Social Services Department.

Skelton, D. (1972), 'Comprehensive geriatric care in general practice' in *Care of the Elderly*, Wessex Regional Hospital Board Report.

Slater, R. (1968), 'The adjustment of residents to old people's homes', *Brit. J. Geriatric Prac.*, September, pp. 299-302.

Stanton, A. H. and Schwartz, M. S. (1954), *The Mental Hospital*, Tavistock.

Storr, A. (1960a), *The Integrity of the Personality*, Heinemann.

Storr, A. (1960b), 'The psychological effects of physical illness', *The Almoner*, vol. 12, no. 12.

Streib, G. F. and Schneider, C. J. (1971), *Retirement in American Society*, Cornell University Press.

Teulings, A. W. M., Jansen, L. C. O. and Verhoeven, W. G. (1973), 'Growth, power structure, and leadership functions in the hospital organisation', *Brit. J. Sociol.*, vol. 24, pp. 490-503.

Topliss, E. P. (1974), 'Organizational change: a case study of a geriatric hospital', *Brit. J. Sociol.*, vol. 25, no. 3.

Townsend, P. (1962), *The Last Refuge*, Routledge & Kegan Paul.

Townsend, P. and Wedderburn, D. (1965), *The Aged in the Welfare State*, Bell.

Tunstall, J. (1966), *Old and Alone*, Routledge & Kegan Paul.

Wager, R. (1972), *Care of the Elderly*, Institute of Municipal Treasurers and Accountants.

Wechsler, D. (1939), *The Measurement of Adult Intelligence*, Williams & Wilkins.

Wechsler, D. (1958), *The Measurement and Appraisal of Adult Intelligence* (4th edn), Baillière, Tindall & Cox.

Whitehead, A. (1970), *In the Service of Old Age*, Penguin Books.

Whitehead, A. (1974), *Psychiatric Disorders in Old Age*, Harvey, Miller & Metcalfe.

Whittingham Report (1972), *Report of the Committee of Inquiry into Whittingham Hospital*, Cmnd 4861, HMSO.

Willcocks, A. J. (ed.) (1975), *The Role of Sheltered Housing in the Care of the Elderly*, Institute of Social Welfare.

Williams, E. I. et al. (1972), 'Sociomedical study of patients over 75 in general practice', *Brit. Med. J.* (ii), pp. 445-8.

Williams Report (1967), *Caring for People: Staffing Residential Homes*, Allen & Unwin.

Williamson, J. et al. (1964), 'Old people at home: their unreported needs', *Lancet*, vol. 1, p. 1117.

Younghusband, E. (1959), Social Work with Individuals, in an essay 'The nature of social work', UN Report 1959, reprinted in A.V.S. Lochhead (ed.) (1968), *A Reader in Social Administration,* Constable.

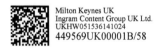